CW01672931

PRACTICAL NUTRITIONAL SUPPORT TECHNIQUES

Second Edition

Alan L. Buchman, MD, MSPH
Northwestern University
Feinberg School of Medicine
Chicago, Ill

SLACK
INCORPORATED
An innovative information, education, and management company
6900 Grove Road • Thorofare, NJ 08086

Copyright © 2004 by SLACK Incorporated

All rights reserved. No part of this book may be reproduced, stored in a retrieval system, or transmitted in any form or by any means, electronic, mechanical, photocopying, recording, or otherwise, without written permission from the publisher, except for brief quotations embodied in critical articles and reviews.

The procedures and practices described in this book should be implemented in a manner consistent with the professional standards set for the circumstances that apply in each specific situation. Every effort has been made to confirm the accuracy of the information presented and to correctly relate generally accepted practices. The author, editor, and publisher cannot accept responsibility for errors or exclusions or for the outcome of the application of the material presented herein. There is no expressed or implied warranty of this book or information imparted by it.

Any review or mention of specific companies or products is not intended as an endorsement by the author or publisher.

The work SLACK Incorporated publishes is peer reviewed. Prior to publication, recognized leaders in the field, educators, and clinicians provide important feedback on the concepts and content that we publish. We welcome feedback on this work.

The first edition of this book was published by Williams & Wilkins in 1997 under the title *Handbook of Nutritional Support.*

Buchman, Alan L.
Practical nutritional support techniques / Alan L. Buchman.-- 2nd ed.
p. ; cm.
Rev. ed. of: Handbook of nutritional support. 1997.
Includes bibliographical references and index.
ISBN 1-55642-628-3 (pbk.)
1. Dietetics--Handbooks, manuals, etc. 2. Nutrition--Handbooks,manuals, etc. 3. Diet therapy--Handbooks, manuals, etc.
[DNLM: 1. Nutritional Support--Handbooks. 2. Diet Therapy--Handbooks. 3. Dietetics--methods--Handbooks. 4. Nutrition Assessment--Handbooks. 5. Nutritional Requirements--Handbooks. WB 39 B919p 2003] I. Buchman, Alan. Handbook of nutritional support. II. Title.
RM217.2 .B78 2003
615.8'54--dc22 2003015309

Printed in the United States of America.

Published by: SLACK Incorporated
6900 Grove Road
Thorofare, NJ 08086 USA
Telephone: 856-848-1000
Fax: 856-853-5991
www.slackbooks.com

Contact SLACK Incorporated for more information about other books in this field or about the availability of our books from distributors outside the United States.

For permission to reprint material in another publication, contact SLACK Incorporated. Authorization to photocopy items for internal, personal, or academic use is granted by SLACK Incorporated provided that the appropriate fee is paid directly to Copyright Clearance Center. Prior to photocopying items, please contact the Copyright Clearance Center at 222 Rosewood Drive, Danvers, MA 01923 USA; phone: 978-750-8400; website: www.copyright.com; email: info@copyright.com.

For further information on CCC, check CCC Online at the following address: http://www.copyright.com.

Last digit is print number: 10 9 8 7 6 5 4 3 2 1

CONTENTS

Acknowledgments

Adult Sections

The main author acknowledges Carrie Kotlar of SLACK Incorporated, who spent countless hours re-typing the manuscript from our first edition, *Handbook of Nutritional Support*, and Charlene Counsellor of SLACK Incorporated for her help in preparing the new edition, *Practical Nutritional Support Techniques*. The author is indebted to Laurie Reyen, RN; Faye Herzog, MD; Donald Yeough, RN; William Guss, PharmD; Reid Nishikowa, PharmD; and Tom Diamantidis, PharmD; for knowledge, nursing protocols, and other materials used in the development of both the *Handbook of Nutritional Support* and *Practical Nutritional Support Techniques*. My nurse, Anita Wallin, RN, and my colleague in the Northwestern Intestinal Rehabilitation Center, Jon Fryer, MD, are to be acknowledged for their incessant help in the care of my patients and in preparation of this book. I also want to thank my colleagues on the Nutrition Support Service of Northwestern Memorial Hospital: Halena Rubin, RPh; Vida Mikalunas, RN; Joan Gerdzos, RN; Mino Minouei, RPh; and Bonnie Kastin, RD; for their care of my patients and for the helpful knowledge they have imparted on me. I am indebted to Patrick Reardon, MD, for the drawings of catheter insertion technique and for Sensormedics who supplied diagrams on indirect calorimetry that were modified for the book. I especially want to thank my mentor, Marvin Ament, MD, for helpful discussions throughout my career and for much of what I have learned. Lastly, but not least, I want to thank my wife Diane for taking care of the house and the dog during all the hours I have spent in the office preparing these books.

Pediatric Section

To Makerere University Medical School in Uganda, East Africa for the excellent exposure to hands-on clinical medicine. To my mentors in nutrition: Virginia Stallings, MD, and Babette Zemel, PhD, for setting a standard of excellence. To Alan Buchman, MD, MSPH, for leading in this joint venture. To Ann Quinn, MS, RD, for extensive review of the several formulas and laying out the data into user-friendly comparison tables. To my parents for nourishing and inspiring me to a life of service, and finally but most appreciably to my wife, Mirika, and children, David, Sam, and Joanna, for being such gifts from God.

About the Authors

Alan L. Buchman, MD, MSPH, became interested in nutrition support as a resident at Cedars Sinai Medical Center. He went on to complete a fellowship in nutrition under Dr. Marvin Ament at UCLA where he also earned his Master of Science degree in Public Health. Following completion of his fellowship in gastroenterology, Dr. Buchman has served on the faculty of the Baylor College of Medicine and the University of Texas at Houston Medical School prior to arriving at Northwestern University. At Northwestern, he is the director of the Inflammatory Bowel Disease Center and co-director of the Intestinal Rehabilitation Center. He is the author of over 100 publications and serves on the editorial boards of many prestigious journals in gastroenterology and nutrition.

Timothy A. Sentongo, MD, is a pediatric gastroenterologist and nutrition specialist. He completed 4 years of combined fellowship training in gastroenterology and nutrition at The Children's Hospital of Philadelphia. He is currently an assistant professor of pediatrics in the Division of Gastroenterology, Hepatology, and Nutrition at Children's Memorial Hospital, Northwestern University, Chicago. He is the director of the Nutrition Assessment Unit and medical director of the Intestinal Failure Program at Children's Memorial Hospital.

INTRODUCTION

This is the second edition of a book that arose out of the need to educate house staff and attending physicians at the Baylor College of Medicine in the practical aspects of nutritional assessment, recognition of the need for nutritional intervention, and planning that intervention with appropriate monitoring for expected outcome. The first edition, the *Handbook of Nutritional Support* appeared in 1997. Readers and reviewers appreciated the "cookbook" approach taken in the book. The current book includes material from the first edition, but has been revised to reflect updated practices. Tables and figures, as well as catheter care procedures, have been updated, and new tables on adult and pediatric enteral formulas have been added. New sections on short bowel syndrome and nutrition in inflammatory bowel disease have also been added. The pediatric chapter has been completely re-written by Dr. Timothy Sentongo.

Since its advent in the late 1960's, nutritional support has become increasingly complex as additional metabolic and technical information has accumulated. It has become exceedingly important for health care providers, including physicians, pharmacists, nurses, dietitians, and trainees, in each of these disciplines engaged in the delivery of nutritional support to become properly educated in its use. That is crucial to achievement of the expected outcomes in a cost-effective manner with minimization of therapy-related complications.

Practical Nutritional Support Techniques is written primarily in an outline format in order to allow for easy accessibility of the information. It is designed as a practical, daily practice guide rather than as a complete referenced textbook. However, more extensive discussion is provided where appropriate. This book is not meant to be an exhaustive text—it only gives the nuts and bolts. References are not provided for all commonly accepted practices; they are only given if the reader might want additional, more detailed information or if the practice is not necessarily common. Special sections for disease-specific nutrition, pregnancy, and commonly encountered conditions in nutritional support (such as short bowel syndrome) are covered.

We are grateful to our patients who have taught us the importance of many of the issues discussed in *Practical Nutritional Support Techniques* and we encourage the health care provider to remember that quality of care is only part of the equation; quality of life for their patient must also be considered.

Alan L. Buchman, MD, MSPH
NORTHWESTERN UNIVERSITY
FEINBERG SCHOOL OF MEDICINE
CHICAGO, ILL

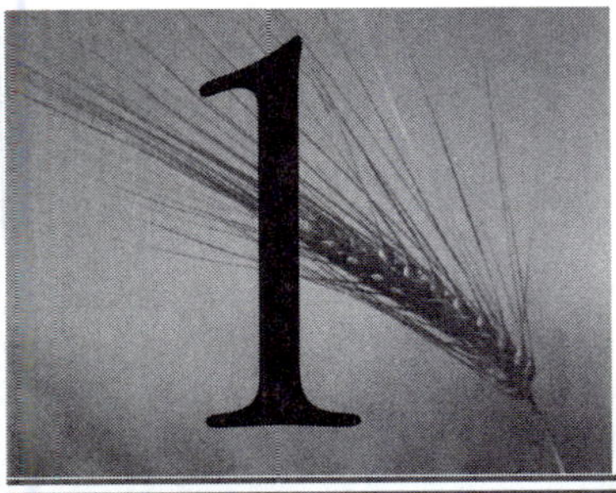

Nutritional Assessment

It is important to realize that no single test can be used as a completely reliable indicator of nutritional status. Proper nutritional assessment should evaluate anthropometric and laboratory data and should include an adequate history and physical examination. Every hospitalized patient should have basic nutritional assessment within 48 hours of admission and every 10 days thereafter.

History and Physical Examination

See Appendix A, Table 1.

History

- Unusual dietary habits
- Medications/vitamin and mineral supplementation
- Change in hair color or texture
- Poor night vision
- Dysgeusia
- Dysphagia/odynophagia
- Abdominal pain-distention
- Diarrhea
- Bone pain
- Muscle pain, cramps, or twitching
- Numbness, parathesias in extremities
- Fatigue
- Diminished mental activity
- Weakness or loss of strength

Physical Examination

- Hair loss, texture
- Keratomalacia
- Cheilosis
- Glossitis
- Red tongue
- Parotid enlargement
- Dentition
- Skin rash, petechiae bruising
- Muscle wasting
- Hepatomegaly
- Edema
- Peripheral neuropathy
- Assess gastrointestinal function: May be affected by malnutrition alone or by primary gastrointestinal disease. Determine the functional status of the gastrointestinal tract, including gastric emptying and intestinal/colonic transit.

ANTHROPOMETRICS

Ideal Body Weight

Further information may be found in Appendix A, Table 2.

ADULT FEMALES

100 lb (45 kg) for the first 60 inches (152 cm) + 5 lbs (2.3 kg) for every inch >60.

ADULT MALES

106 lb (48 kg) for the first 60 inches (152 cm) + 6 lbs (2.7 kg) for every inch >60.

Percent of Usual or Ideal Body Weight

Significant potential for malnutrition:

>5% weight loss in 1 month
>7.5% weight loss in 3 months
>10% weight loss in 6 months

Preferred Body Weight For Obese Patients

$$(ABW - IBW)(0.25) + IBW$$

ABW = actual body weight
IBW = ideal body weight

	Usual or IBW (%)
Mild malnutrition	85 to 90
Moderate malnutrition	75 to 84
Severe malnutrition	<74

The minimal survival weight is 48% to 55% of IBW.[1]

Adjusted Body Weight for Amputation

Measured weight - % amputation

Corrections for Amputation	
Entire arm	6.5%
Upper arm	3.5%
Hand	0.8%
Forearm with hand	3.1%
Forearm without hand	2.5%
Entire leg	18.6%
Foot	1.8%

Mid-Arm Muscle Circumference

Mid-arm muscle circumference (MAMC) (cm) = Mid-arm circumference (MAC) (cm) – 3.14 (triceps skinfold in cm)

- Assess skeletal mass
- Compare with normal values (Appendix A, Table 3)
  - <5th%—depletion
  - 5th% to 25th%—at risk for depletion
  - <85th%—at risk for obesity
- Not routinely used because it is operator-dependent (variability); unreliable indicator of short-term response to nutritional therapy. Primarily for use in population studies.

Muscle Function

Muscle function testing is not usually useful as an initial screening tool, but may be useful in serial assessments. Improvements in hand grip strength measured by dynamometry or respiratory muscle strength (peak inspiratory and expiratory pressures) are useful (Appendix A, Tables 4 and 5).

Triceps Skinfold Thickness

- Assess fat stores
- Compare with normal values (Appendix A, Tables 6, 7, and 8)
- Not routinely used because it is operator-dependent (variability); unreliable indicator of short-term response to nutritional therapy. Primarily for use in population studies.

Methods of Measuring Skinfolds and Circumferences

See Figure 3-3.

Skinfolds

1. Arrive at the anatomic site as defined (the midpoint between the acromial and olecranon process of the scapula and the ulna, respectively). The arm should hang relaxed at the patient's side.
2. Lift the skin and fat layer from the underlying tissue by grasping the tissue with the thumb and forefinger.
3. Apply calipers about 1 cm distal from the thumb and forefinger, midway between the apex and the base of the skinfold.
4. Continue to support the skinfold with the thumb and forefinger for the duration of the measurement.
5. After 2 to 3 seconds of caliper application, read skinfold to the nearest 0.5 mm.
6. Measurements are then made in triplicate until readings within ± 1.0 mm; results are then averaged.

Circumferences

1. The tape should be maintained in a horizontal position touching the skin and following the contours of the limb, but not compressing the underlying tissue.
2. Measurements should be made to the nearest millimeter, in triplicate, as previously described for skinfolds.

Laboratory Measurements

Nitrogen Balance

- Often helpful in determining whether sufficient protein and/or calories are being provided.

$$N(g) = \frac{g\ protein/d}{6.25}$$

The average protein is approximately 15% nitrogen, hence 6.25 is used as the denominator.

To calculate nitrogen output:

- Use 24-hour total urine nitrogen (TUN) or urine urea nitrogen (UUN). (TUN is preferable.)

  - UUN represents, on the average, only 80% to 90% of TUN, although the range can be as great as 12% to 112%. This may result in variations of up to 12 g.[2]
  - Increased nonurea nitrogen (including uric acid, ammonia, creatinine, and other minor compounds) loss may occur during "stress," especially in major burns[3] or a change in hydration status.
  - Avoid pH adjustments and heating of urine samples because this may lead to falsely low TUN.[4]
- Daily fecal N losses in patients without malabsorption or protein-losing enteropathy during parenteral nutrition range between 0.3 to 0.8 g/day or approximately 8 mg/kg/day.
- Integumental losses, in the absence of large wounds or burns, range between 7 mg/kg/day for women and 8 mg/kg/day for men.[5]

$$\text{Nitrogen balance} = N_{intake(I)} - N_{output\ (0)}$$
or
$$N_I - (UUN + 4)$$

- For anabolism, +N balance of at least 4 to 6 g is required.
- Achievement of positive N balance requires not only sufficient protein or amino acids, but adequate calories as well.
- N retention does not necessarily indicate effective N utilization.

Indirect Calorimetry

- Measures the basal energy expenditure (BEE) required to fuel basic life functions at rest in a neutral thermic environment, 10 or more hours after eating.
- Helpful in estimating caloric requirements, especially in patients who are significantly underweight or overweight (with significant fluid retention) or significantly catabolic.
- BEE is estimated from known values of heat produced by the combustion of carbohydrate, fat, and protein and measurement of inspired O_2 and expired CO_2 using the Weir equation.[6]

$$\text{kcal/d} = (3.941 \times \dot{V}O_2\ [\text{L/day}]) + (1.106 \times \dot{V}CO_2\ [\text{L/day}]) - (2.17 \times \text{TUN}\ [\text{g/day}])$$

$\dot{V}O_2 = O_2$ consumption

$\dot{V}CO_2 = CO_2$ production

- Most typically utilized in an open-circuit system in which patient breathes either ambient or oxygen-enriched air (via a ventilator or non-air leak face mask).

MECHANISM

In the nonventilated patient a clear plastic hood, through which a stream of room air flows, is placed over the patient's head (Figure 1-1). Alternatively, a mouthpiece (into which the patient inspires and expires) with a noseclip to avoid nasal inspiration/expiration can be used. For the ventilated patient, a vacuum line is interposed between the endotracheal tube and ventilator tube (Figure 1-2). The expired gas is diluted and removed through the expiratory port of the hood or mouthpiece. The diluted air is passed through a volume-measuring device (for measurement of minute ventilation), through a mixing chamber (to achieve a steady concentration of inspired gases), and then through O_2 and CO_2 analyzers. In the ventilated patient, inspired and expired gases are sampled continuously at a constant rate.

O_2 consumption and CO_2 production are calculated from measurements of inspired and expired gas and from minute ventilation. The difference in gas concentration between room air and exhaled air is multiplied by the gas flow rate through the system. The process is similar in a ventilated patient, except that a vacuum line is interposed. O_2 and CO_2 measurements are weighted according to the corresponding flow rate measured simultaneously by the pneumotach. A phase delay ensures that gas and flow measurements are appropriately matched.

PROCEDURE

- Usually requires about 30 minutes to perform, including a 10-minute equilibration period in which the patient is allowed to become accustomed to the hood or mouthpiece/noseclip system to exclude a hyperventilation artifact and to allow for achievement of a steady state.
- Patient should be resting, but not asleep during the test period.
- There should be no interruption, such as medication dosing, eating, phlebotomy, or ventilator adjustments during the test period.
- Valid gas measurement cannot be obtained for patients who are receiving supplemental oxygen via non-airtight facemask, nasal cannula, or >60% FiO_2. Even small fluctuations in inspired O_2 tension, commonly encountered in many mechanical ventilator systems, can markedly alter O_2 consumption measurement, especially when a high FiO_2 is used.
- $\dot{V}O_2$ is usually 3 to 4 ml/min/kg in normal subjects, so any outlying values should be evaluated. For example, a patient in extreme pain or with head trauma who is hyperventilating may have a $\dot{V}O_2$ of 5 to 7 ml/min/kg. Incorrect values may be caused by leaks, inaccurate volume measurements, or unstable gas analyzers.
- Consult individual factory technical manuals for information and other technical problems or calibration of the metabolic cart.
- Perform after a minimum of 6 hours fasting (preferably 8 to 12 hours). It is unnecessary to discontinue continuous feeding (enteral or parenteral), but keep in mind the resting energy expenditure (REE) will then include the thermogenic effect of food. The thermogenic effect of food is on the order of 10%,[7] although a range of 5% to 30% has been reported.

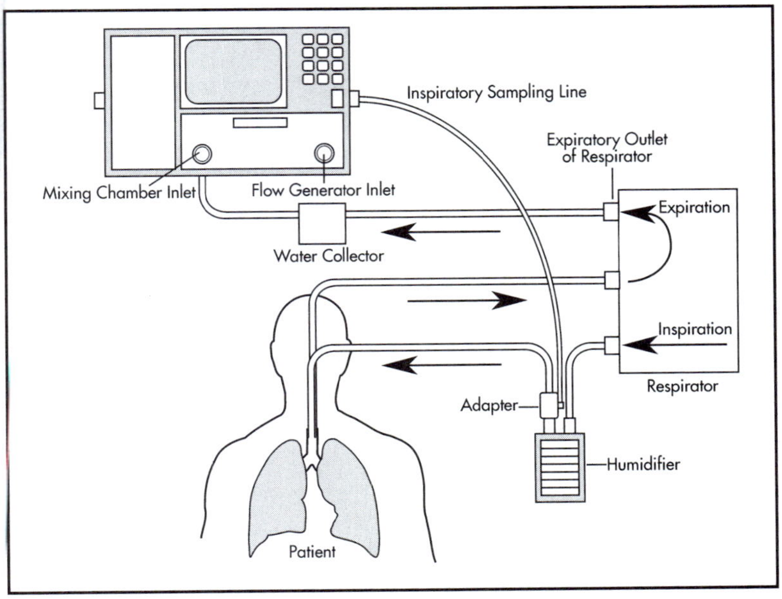

Figure 1-1. Indirect calorimetry respiratory measurements for ventilated patient. Illustration by Barbie Minnick.

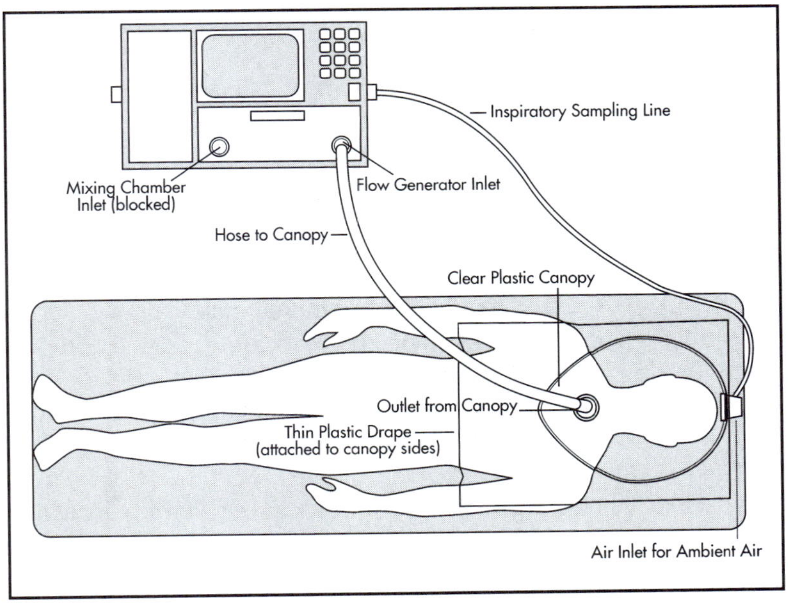

Figure 1-2. Indirect calorimetry canopy measurements with room air. Illustration by Barbie Minnick.

- Hypo- or hypermetabolism occur when measured REE varies more than 10% from that predicted using the Harris Benedict equations.
- Total energy expenditure includes an activity factor, and the thermogenic response to food (either parenteral or enteral), and is thought to add approximately 20% to the REE for patients undergoing "usual" hospital treatment. Additional activity such as intense rehabilitation will increase caloric demands, while a comatose patient will expend little energy for activity. The only rules are to use common sense, follow response to nutritional therapy, and repeat the indirect calorimetry at regular intervals if necessary.

Factors Affecting REE	
Height and weight	Pain
Age	Fever/hypothermia
Sex	Thermogenic effect of food
Medications	Sleep/awake

High REE	*Low REE*
Caffeine	Beta blockers
Aspirin	Alpha blockers
Epinephrine	Anesthesia

Situations in Which Metabolic Measurements May Be Unreliable

- FiO_2>60%
- Hyperventilation
- Poor patient cooperation (agitated or sleeping)
- Bronchopleural fistula
- Trachea cuff leak
- Positive-end expiratory pressure (PEEP), peak expiratory flow rate (PEFR)
- Tremor, seizures

Respiratory Quotient

- Calculated by determining the ratio of expired CO_2 to inspired O_2.

Respiratory quotient (RQ) >1.0	Usually reflects nonsteady state, hyperventilation, or overfeeding
RQ = 1.0	Carbohydrate oxidation
RQ = 0.85	Mixed substrate "oxidation"
RQ = 0.70	Fax oxidation
RQ = 1.0 to 1.2	Lipogenesis
RQ = 0.67	Alcohol and ketone metabolism

- It is important to note whether the RQ is within physiologic range (0.7 to 1.3) and consistent with the patient's nutritional intake. For example, the RQ should be 0.7 to 0.8 (consistent with fat oxidation) in a patient whose sole nutritional intake has been D_5W for a week. Therefore, an RQ of >1.0 should be viewed with suspicion in such a patient.
- Errors may have been caused by technical problems (eg, hyperventilation because the patient received an injection during the gas measurement), the unrecorded administration, or a large dextrose load.
- RQ may vary during hemo- or peritoneal dialysis.[8]

Factors Increasing RQ		
Hyperventilation	Overfeeding/lipogenesis	
Metabolic acidosis	Exercise	Calibration errors or leaks in the metabolic cart

Visceral Proteins

Albumin

Normal (3.5 to 5.0 g/dL)
Mildly depleted (3.0 to 3.5 g/dL)

Moderately depleted (2.5 to 3.0 g/dL)
Severely depleted (<2.5 g/dL)

- Poor indicator of short-term changes in visceral protein status and may be unreliable in some medical conditions.[9]
- Non-nutritional factors may elevate albumin concentration (eg, albumin infusion, dehydration, renal failure and suppressed-in hepatic failure, anabolic steroids).[10]
- Non-nutritional factors may depress albumin concentration (eg, pregnancy, severe burns, protein-losing enteropathy, nephrotic syndrome, edema, hepatic insufficiency, neoplastic disease, severe infections, trauma, or post surgery).[10]

Pre-Albumin

Normal (18 to 24 mg/dL)
Mildly deplete (16 to 18 mg/dL)
Moderately depleted (14 to 16 mg/dL)
Severely depleted (<14 mg/dL)

- More sensitive marker than albumin for assessing rapid nutritional changes, although subject to similar non-nutritional factors.
- May be elevated in renal failure and suppressed in hepatic failure.
- Pre-albumin and nitrogen balance measurement are the preferred parameters in the assessment of total body protein status.

Transferrin

Normal (200 to 250 mg/dL)
Mildly depleted (170 to 200 mg/dL)
Moderately depleted (140 to 170 mg/dL)
Severely depleted (<140 mg/dL)

- May be elevated due to iron deficiency anemia, as an acute phase reactant, during pregnancy, or during the use of oral contraceptives.
- May be suppressed-in renal and hepatic failure despite adequate protein status.
- Although a significant relationship exists between serum transferrin concentration and nutritional status, the variation in concentration may lend a greater usefulness in population studies rather than in the individual patient.[11]

Retinol-Binding Protein

- Half life is 12 hours. This is too short for practical value and has no advantages over pre-albumin.

Insulin-Like Growth Factor-1

- Investigational[12]

Immune Function

Total Lymphocyte Count

Normal (1600 to 4000 per mm^3)
Mildly depleted (1200 to 1600 m^3)
Moderately depleted (800 to 1200 per m^3)
Severely depleted (<800 per m^3)

- May be depressed by non-nutritional factors including chemotherapy, radiation therapy, glucocorticoids, and viral infections.

DELAYED HYPERSENSITIVITY SKIN TESTS

- Commonly used antigens include mumps, trichophyton, candida, tetanus, and intermediate strength purified protein derivative (PPD). A 5-mm response or greater at 24 to 48 hours is considered a positive response.
- May be affected by non-nutritional factors including corticosteroids, T-cell deficiency, cancer, or immunosuppressive medications.

REFERENCES

1. University of Minnesota Laboratory of Physiological Hygiene. *The Biology of Starvation,* 1950.
2. Konstantinides FN, Konstantinides NN, Li JC, et al. Urinary urea nitrogen: too insensitive for calculating nitrogen balance studies in surgical clinical nutrition. *JPEN.* 1991:15:189-193.
3. Bell SJ, Molner JA, Kraske WS. Prediction of total urinary nitrogen from urea nitrogen of burned patients. *J Am Diet Assoc.* 1985;85:1100-1104.
4. Konstantinides FN, Maga VK, Herman BA, et al. Routine laboratory preparation of twenty-four-hour urine samples for nitrogen determinations induces false low total urinary nitrogen (TUN) levels. *JPEN.* 1992;16:33S.
5. Calloway DH, Odell AC, Margen S. Sweat and miscellaneous nitrogen losses in human balance studies. *J Nutr.* 1971;101:775-786.
6. Weir JB. New methods for calculating metabolic rate with special reference to protein metabolism. *J Physiol.* 1949;109:1-9.
7. Elwyn DH, Kinney JM, Askanazi J. Energy expenditure in surgical patients. *Surg Clin North Am.* 1981;61:545-549.
8. Sigler MH, Skutches CL, Teehan BP, et al. Acetate and energy metabolism during hemodialysis. *Kidney Intl Sup.* 1983;24:597-610.
9. Socolow EL, Woeber KA, Purdy RH, et al. Preparation of I131-labeled human serum prealbumin and its metabolism in normal and sick patients. *J Clin Invest.* 1965;44:1600-1609.
10. Ingenbleek Y, van den Schrieck HG, de Nayer P, et al. Albumin, transferrin and the thyroxine-binding prealbumin/retinal-binding protein (TBPA-RBP) complex in assessment of malnutrition. *Clin Chem Acta.* 1975;63:61-67.
11. Ryan JA Jr, Page CP. Intra-jejunal feeding: development and current status. *JPEN.* 1984;8:523-528.
12. Donahue SP, Phillips LS. Response of IGF-1 to nutritional support in malnourished hospital patients: a possible indicator of short-term changes in nutritional status. *Am J Clin Nutr.* 1989;50:962-969.

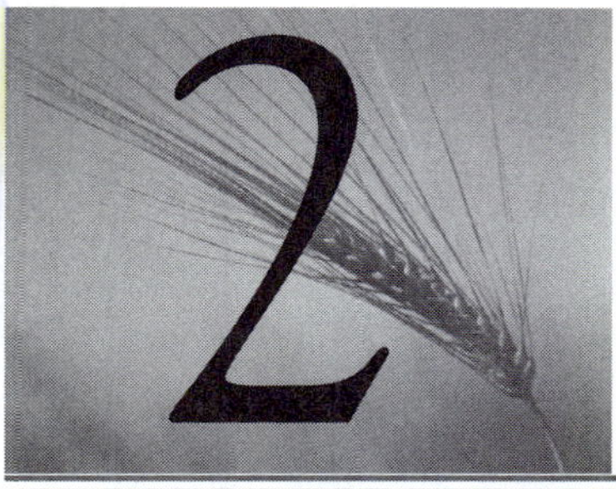

Nutritional Requirements

Fluid Requirements

Maintenance

1500 ml + 20 ml/kg for every kg > 20 kg

- Increases by 10% for every 1°C of fever.
- May be decreased significantly in cirrhosis, congestive heart failure, pulmonary edema, acute respiratory distress syndrome (ARDS), or renal failure.

Replacement Fluid

- Extraneous fluid losses (eg, nasogastric or enteric suction, biliary or fistula drainage diarrhea or emesis) should be replaced with a separate intravenous solution in amounts equal to measured losses every 8 hours. Fluid retention may also occur during total parenteral nutrition (TPN). Weight gain of >1 to 2 kg/wk is probably related to fluid retention.
- Avoid the use of TPN to replace extraneous fluid and electrolyte losses because of the significant extra expense. Replace with common intravenous electrolyte solutions when possible.
- See Appendix A, Table 14 for body fluid electrolyte concentrations.

Caloric Requirements

Actual caloric requirements can only be estimated in the absence of direct calorimetry. The formulas shown and indirect calorimetry are helpful in making the appropriate estimations.

Harris Benedict Equation

- Estimates basal metabolic rate (BMR).

Males: 66.47 + 13.75 (weight, kg) + 5 (height, cm) – 6.76 (age, yr)
Females: 655.1 + 9.56 (weight, kg) + 1.85 (height, cm) – 4.68 (age, yr)

- Multiply result by 1.2 to 1.5 "activity" factors to account for physical activity and disease stress.
- Derived from studies on young healthy adults, so it is often inaccurate in the hospital setting, especially in critically ill patients. For instance, when the REE is measured in trauma, or with infected or mechanically ventilated patients using indirect calorimetry, values of 70% to 140% of those predicted using the Harris Benedict equation have been described.[1,2] Studies in acutely ill surgical patients show that the Harris Benedict equation may overestimate caloric requirements by an average of 59%.[3] Each degree (°C) increase in body temperature increases the REE by 7% to 13%.[4-6] Mechanical ventilation and medication such as barbiturates, muscle relaxants such as curare and pancuronium, and beta blockers such as propranolol may decrease metabolic rate. Metabolic rate is usually increased significantly in patients with major burns because significant energy must be used to maintain body temperature. However, the REE usually declines during convalescence. Care must be taken not to undernourish or overfeed patients.

Indirect Calorimetry

- Measures REE.
- Add ~20% for activity.

Caloric Requirements by Ideal Body Weight or Preferred Body Weight

- Maintenance (25 to 30 kcal/kg)

  REBUILD LEAN BODY MASS (35 TO 40 KCAL/KG)

- In patients who are severely underweight, REE is often depressed and actual body weight should be used in preference to IBW in the initial days of nutritional support to avoid refeeding syndrome (hypophosphatemia).

Calorie:Nitrogen Ratio

- Sufficient non-protein calories (ie, dextrose, lipid) must be administered to enable the efficient use of protein synthesis and to prevent the catabolism of skeletal muscle and exogenous amino acids for use as a calorie support with subsequent development of kwashiorkor. Protein provides 5.65 kcal/g. However, when the water dilution of protein and the energy lost in the form of urea are considered, protein supplies only 1 kcal/g. Therefore, protein becomes a poor and expensive glucose source when sufficient dextrose calories are not provided.

- The optimal non-protein calorie:nitrogen ratio is 150: to 200:1.
- See Appendix A, Table 9 for ratios in standard TPN solution.

Protein Requirements

Protein requirements can only be estimated in the absence of nitrogen balance determination.

- 0.6 to 0.8 g/kg/day in healthy humans.
- 0.8 to 1.0 g/kg/day in hospitalized patients.
- 1.1 to 1.5 g/kg/day for protein repletion.
- >1.5 g/kg/day only in severe burns and protein losing enteropathy. Excess protein will not result in greater tissue synthesis.
- 0.55 g/kg/day minimum in renal failure or hepatic failure in the absence of dialysis.[7]
- Add 6 to 9 g/day for hemodialysis, including CHD and CVVHD (1.0 to 1.2 g/kg/d).[8,9]
- Add 12 to 16 g/day for peritoneal dialysis (1.2 to 1.4 g/kg/d).[10-12]

Specialized Amino Acid Products

See Appendix A, Table 23 for product composition.

Branched Chain Amino Acids

High Branched Chain Formula

The high branched chain (HBC) formula is possibly of benefit in severely catabolic patients with multiple trauma, sepsis, or multiorgan failure syndrome and lactic acidosis and hyperglycemia. Clinical efficacy has not been demonstrated. Therefore, this formulation should not be used outside of a research protocol.

Elevated Branched Chain /Low Aromatic Amino Acid Formula

The use of this formula is predicated by the false neurotransmitter theory of James et al[13] and the observation that serum ammonia concentration is often elevated in hepatic encephalopathy. The false neurotransmitter theory assumes that the imbalance between plasma elevated branched chain amino acid (BCAA)/(leucine, isoleucine, and valine) and low aromatic amino acid (AAA) (tyrosine, phenylalanine, and tryptophan) leads to an increased influx of the AAA into the brain. BCAA and AAA compete for the same amino acid transporter across the blood-brain barrier (BBB). Relative plasma concentration gradients determine those amino acids preferentially transported across the BBB. The relative increase in plasma AAA leads to increased AAA across the BBB and into the brain. The excessive amounts of these AAA are the precursors of "false neurotransmitters" such as octopamine and B-phenylethanolamine, which are thought to precipitate hepatic coma.

The therapeutic approach of using a high BCAA- or low AAA-containing formula is an attempt to normalize the relative plasma amino acid concentrations. In addition, high BCAA/low AAA formulas provide substrates that bind ammonia:

valine → succinate → a-ketoglutarate
glutamine → glutamate
↓
NH3

Leucine, in particular, stimulates protein synthesis and thereby possibly inhibits protein and peripheral muscle catabolism, thus generating less ammonia.

Although theoretically attractive, the clinical efficacy of high BCAA/low AAA formulas have not been conclusively demonstrated. Therefore, and because of the extra expense of this formulation, clear outcome goals in a specified time trial are necessary for its use; if efficacy is demonstrated in a given patient, the formula may be continued until it has been determined that the patient had improved to the point where use of standard amino acid formulas might be tolerated.

Renal Formula

This formulation consists of only essential amino acids. Histidine is considered an essential amino acid in renal failure. While theoretically beneficial, clinical studies have demonstrated no improvement in morbidity or mortality and no consistent decrease in urea generation when compared with standard amino acid solutions in equivalent amounts. At best, only small metabolic improvements may be noted. Therefore, this formula should not be used outside of a research protocol.[14,15] There may be benefit from using specialized renal formulas during continuous arterial venous hyperfiltration (CAVH) when nitrogenous wastes are not removed. However, these formulas have not been studied in randomized-controlled trials during CAVH.

Fat Requirements

The minimum fat content of the diet is 2% to 4% of total calories consisting of linoleic acid. That is to prevent essential fatty acid deficiency (EFAD). Decreased serum linoleic acid concentration, an increase in ratio of 5:8:11 eicosatrienoic acid to arachidonic acid to >0.4. Increased palmitoleic and oleic acid concentrations may also be found. Scaly skin rash, hair loss, hepatomegaly, anemia, thrombocytopenia, osteoporosis, and decreased wound healing may occur. Most lipid emulsions are typically 50% linoleic acid. Medium chain triglycerides (MCT) do not provide essential fats. Linolenic acid has not been conclusively demonstrated to be essential in humans because only a single case report of a child developing a neuropathy associated with linolenic acid deficiency has been reported. Biochemical evidence of EFAD may occur within 2 weeks of the provision of lipid-free TPN, although clinical deficiency does not develop for about 6 weeks.

Electrolyte, Vitamin, and Trace Element Requirements

Requirements may vary depending on underlying pathology and the need to replace deficient states or to prevent toxicity. For most patients receiving parenteral nutrition, standard electrolyte, vitamin, and trace element solutions will provide daily patient needs if adequate calories are infused (see Appendix A, Tables 10, 26, and 27). Likewise, most enteral products are designed to meet the recommended dietary allowance (RDA) for electrolytes, vitamins, and trace elements if adequate amounts to provide optimal caloric intake are provided. It is important to include electrolyte content such as sodium and potassium bound to medication in the calculation of daily intake (see Appendix A, Tables 31 through 34).

Electrolyte Abnormalities

- May result from inadequate replacement of body losses (see Appendix A, Table 14).
- As protein synthesis occurs with refeeding, potassium and phosphorus requirements will increase.
- Extreme hyperglycemia will cause a pseudohyponatremia.
- Increased endogenous or exogenous insulin will cause a decrease in serum potassium and possibly magnesium.
- See Appendix A, Table 15 for signs and symptoms of electrolyte abnormalities.

Trace Element Abnormalities

- May result from inadequate replacement of body losses (eg, zinc and selenuim lost in diarrhea) or excessive replacement (eg, copper during severe cholestasis).
- See Appendix A, Table 16 for signs and symptoms of trace element abnormalities.

Vitamin Abnormalities

- Unusual.
- May result from excessive replacement during states of inadequate metabolism/excretion (eg, vitamin A in renal failure).
- See Appendix A, Table 17 for signs and symptoms of vitamin deficiency/toxicity.
- Required water soluble vitamins in humans include thiamine (B_1), riboflavin (B_2), niacin (B_3), pantothenic acid (B_5), pyridoxin (B_6), cyanocobalamin (B_{12}), folic acid ascorbic acid (C), and biotin.
- Required fat soluble vitamins include retinol (A), calciferol (D), tocopherol (E), and phytonadione (K).

REFERENCES

1. Carlson M, Nordenstrom J, Hedenstierna G. Clinical implications of continuous measurement of energy expenditure in mechanically ventilated patients. *Clin Nutr.* 1984;3:103-110.
2. Weissman C, Kemper M, Askenazi J, et al. Resting metabolic rate of the critically ill patient: measured versus predicted. *Anesthesiology.* 1986;64:673-679.
3. Mann S, Westenskow DR, Houtchens BA. Measured and predicted caloric expenditure in the acutely ill. *Crit Care Med.* 1985;13:173-177.
4. Paige DM. *Clinical Nutrition.* 2nd ed. St. Louis: Mosby; 1988:363.
5. Shils ME, Olson JA, Shike M. *Modern Nutrition.* 8th ed. Philadelphia: Lee and Febiger; 1988:826.
6. Kiney JM, Furst P, Elwyn OH, et al. The Intensive Care Patients. In: Kinney JM, Jeejeebhoy K, Hill GL, Owen OE, eds. *Nutrition and Metabolism in Patient Care.* Philadelphia: WB Saunders; 1988:658.
7. Eastwood M. Dietary fiber and the risks of cancer. *Nutr Rev.* 1987;39:193.
8. Kopple JD, Swendseid ME, Shinaberger JH, et al. The free end band amino acids removed by henodialysis. *Trans Am Soc Artif Int Organ.* 1973:4:309.
9. Davies Sp. Amino acid clearance and daily losses in patients with acute renal failure treated by continuous arteriovenous hemodialysis. *Crit Care Med.* 1991;19:1510.
10. Berlyne GM, Lee HA, Giordano C, et al. Amino acid loss in peritoneal dialysis. *Lancet.* 1967:1339-1341.
11. Kopple JD, Monteon FJ, Shaib JK. Effect of energy intake on nitrogen metabolism in non-dialyzed patients with chronic renal failure. *Kidney Int.* 1986;29:734.
12. Blumenkrantz MJ, Kopple JD, Moran JK, et al. Metabolic balance studies and dietary protein requirements in patients undergoing continuous ambulatory peritoneal dialysis. *Kidney Int.* 1982;21:849.
13. James JH, Ziparo V, Jeppsson B, et al. Hyperammonemia, plasma amino acid imbalance, and blood-brain amino acid transport; a unified theory of portal-systemic encephalopathy. *Lancet.* 1979;2:772.
14. Feinstein EI, Blumenkrantz. Clinical and metabolic responses to parenteral nutrition in acute renal failure: A controlled double-blind study. *Medicine.* 1981;60:124.
15. Druml W. Nutritional support in acute renal failure. *Clin Nutr.* 1993;12:196.

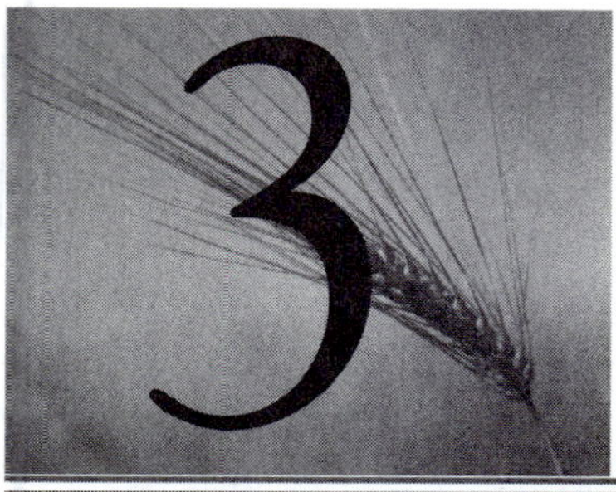

Parenteral Nutrition

Indications

In general, total parenteral nutrition (TPN) is indicated if the small intestine is dysfunctional, obstructed, or inaccessible; or the colon is severely dysfunctional or obstructed; and the condition is expected to continue a minimum of 7 days.

Specific Indications

1. *Intractable vomiting*—eg, severe acute pancreatitis, hyperemesis gravidarum, chemotherapy.
2. *Severe diarrhea*—(>500 ml/day stool) or malabsorption (eg, severe, acute flare of inflammatory bowel disease, graft versus host disease, severe sprue or sprue-like conditions), short bowel syndrome (<50 to 60 cm of remaining bowel), radiation enteritis with weight loss.
3. *Severe mucositis/esophagitis*—eg, chemotherapy, graft versus host disease.
4. *Ileus*—eg, severe trauma/major abdominal surgery or pseudo-obstruction, when enteral nutrition, including feeding jejunostomy cannot be used for at least 7 days.
5. *Small bowel or colon obstruction*—eg, cancer, adhesions, infectious, pseudo-obstruction.
6. *"Bowel Rest"*—eg, enterocutaneous or entero-enteric fistula, anastomotic leak, Crohn's disease of small intestine.
7. *Preoperative*—eg, only in cases of severe malnutrition, otherwise surgery should not be delayed.
   A. *Intraoperative* parenteral nutrition is relatively contraindicated; there is no demonstrated efficacy, and should intraoperative fluid resuscitation be required, the risk of inadvertently increasing the parenteral nutrition (PN) infusion rate could have potentially serious ramifications. Severe metabolic and/or electrolyte disturbances may occur rapidly in the perioperative period.

8. Parenteral nutrition is *not* indicated in patients who have a gastrointestinal tract capable of adequate nutrient absorption, whenever parenteral duration is expected to be less than 7 days, in mildly malnourished preoperative patients, in patients in whom parenteral nutrition is not desired by the patient or legal guardian, or in whom the disease prognosis is not improved by the use of parenteral nutrition. On the other hand, the nutritional assessment for nutritional support should be considered within the first 24 hours; do not wait 7 days.

Central Parenteral Nutrition

- The high osmolality (>900 mOsm) of most central parenteral nutrition (CPN) solutions requires administration into large veins with high blood flow in order to avoid phlebitis. The catheter tip should rest in the superior or inferior vena cava.
- To limit the risk of infection, a central venous catheter inserted solely for the use of CPN should be used.

Peripheral Parenteral Nutrition

- Peripheral parenteral nutrition (PPN) should be provided to patients who require only short-term therapy (<7 to 10 days) and can meet some but not all of their nutritional requirements via enteral means. This therapy may provide for some protein sparing.
- Because the solutions are hypertonic, thrombophlebitis of the site of administration is inevitable. Never use dextrose solutions of greater than 10% concentration or 900 mOsm (Appendix A, Table 19).
- Hydrocortisone 10 mg and heparin 1000 units/l may prevent thrombophlebitis.[1,2] There are rare reports of heparin-induced thrombocytopenia.
- Hospital policy often precludes administration of intravenous medications into the same peripheral vein as parenteral nutrition known to cause phlebitis (acyclovir, aminoglycosides, amphotericin, erythromycin, high dose penicillins, phenytoin, potassium, vancomycin).

Intradialytic Parenteral Nutrition

- Intradialytic parenteral nutrition (IDPN) is indicated only in patients who are receiving chronic hemodialysis, have poor oral intake, and can not be enterally fed or provided with CPN. Medicare regulations enacted in June 1987 are stringent on the proper indications. The medical record must demonstrate the patient has poor dietary intake, has lost >10% of dry weight, has fat and peripheral muscle wasting, depressed serum albumin, in addition to one or more of the diagnoses listed under indications for PN.
- IDPN is safe[3] if a moderate infusion rate is maintained and proper monitoring is performed. Typical infusion is a single liter and includes approximately 7 kcal/kg from dextrose, 1.6 g/kg of lipid emulsion, and 0.22 g/kg amino acids. The rate should be initiated at no more than 150 ml/hr to avoid profound hyperglycemia. The rate is then gradually increased so that the full liter can be infused during a 4-hour dialysis. The increased lipid as a percentage of

total calories may be helpful in avoiding the hyperglycemia, although large triglyceride loads may not be handled well either. The superiority of an essential amino acid-containing formula over a mixed essential/nonessential amino acid-containing formula has not been demonstrated.[4] Blood glucose monitoring should be frequent during the infusion and at 30 and 60 minutes after the infusion to detect reactive hypoglycemia, which may be more life threatening than the hyperglycemia. If possible, some sweetened orange juice or other simple carbohydrate beverage should be provided 20 to 30 minutes after the infusion.

Contraindications

PN may not be appropriate in hemodynamically unstable patients including those with hypovolemia, cardiogenic or septic shock; patients with severe pulmonary edema or fluid overload; patients with anuria without dialysis; or patients with profound metabolic or electrolyte disturbances. Concentrated PN may be required for patients with overhydration.

Components of Parenteral Nutrition

Central Venous Catheter

See Appendix A, Table 18.

- Catheter tip should rest in the superior or inferior vena cava and be documented by radiography before initiation of infusion.
- Double and triple lumen short-term catheters may be used if a dedicated PN line is unavailable. However, multi-lumen catheters carry a higher rate of sepsis than single lumen catheters. If multi-lumen catheters must be used, a designated PN port should be used. A pulmonary artery catheter (Swan-Ganz) is a violated line and should not be used for PN. Intrusion of a central venous catheter should be permitted only under emergency conditions (eg, CPR). A catheter lumen reserved for PN should not be used for central venous pressure (CVP) monitoring, blood infusion, or drug therapy.
- The use of routine line changes/replacement is controversial. It remains unclear as to whether routine line change or replacement is associated with decreased infection risk. There are mechanical risks associated with replacement.[5,6]

Catheter Types

Short-Term Catheters	*Long-Term Catheters*
Triple, double, single lumen (eg, Arrow Cath, Cook Cath)	Tunneled silastic, single and double lumen (eg, Hickman, Broviac)
Cordis	Percutaneous inserted central catheter (PICC lines)
Swan-Ganz (pulmonary artery catheters)	Subcutaneous infusion ports
Arterial lines	

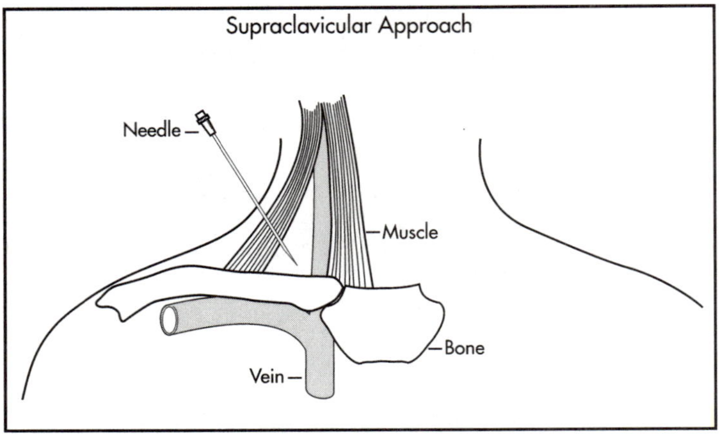

Figure 3-1. The subclavian vein is the preferred route for central venous access. Illustration by Barbie Minnick.

CATHETER INSERTION

Site Choice

The subclavian vein is the preferred route for central venous access for TPN (Figure 3-1). This site allows for access to the central circulation and provides an immobile area for catheter fixation. This not only makes it more comfortable for the patient, but the broad, flat surface allows for placement of a truly occlusive dressing. This may be difficult to achieve in some patients.

The internal jugular vein is the next most frequently accessed site. The neck is much more mobile, however, and lines placed at these sites are more uncomfortable for the patient. The rounded surface of the neck with its muscular contours makes achieving a truly occlusive dressing more difficult as well.

The femoral vein site may be associated with an increased incidence of infection. The skin puncture site is frequently at the groin crease, where the skin flora has a greater concentration of potentially pathogenic organisms. This is a warm, moist area with a great deal of movement. This makes maintenance of an occlusive dressing very difficult. Infusion of concentrated solutions into these veins may lead to iliofemoral vein thrombosis with its subsequent risk of pulmonary embolism. This site should almost never be accessed for TPN if other more preferable sites are available.

Technique

TRIPLE-LUMEN CATHETER

- Informed consent.
- The operator should don cap, mask, sterile gown, and sterile gloves.
- Place patient in Trendelenburg position with head turned away from the catheterization site.
- Prep skin with povidone-iodine or 2% chlorhexidine from the sternum to the lateral edge of the chest and from the jaw line to 8 to 10 cm below the clavicle.
- Use patient's nondominant side if possible.
- Use sterile towel or drapes to provide a sterile field.
- Determine the length of the catheter to be inserted so that the tip resides within the superior vena cava (SVC) if possible (never in the heart). The external

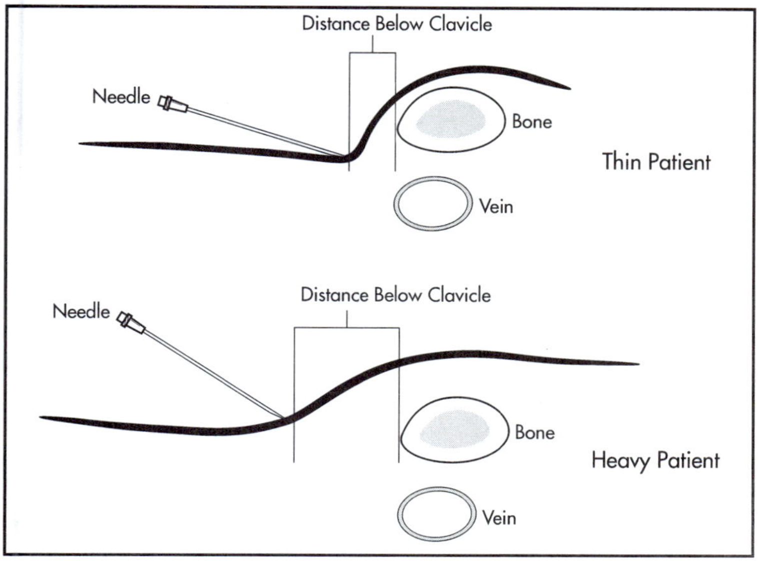

Figure 3-2. Distance below clavicle. Illustration by Barbie Minnick.

marker for the junction of the SVC and the right atrium is at the Louis Angle, where the manubrium and sternal body meet. Then place the catheter along the track of the vein until the guidewire is met. The distance along the catheter may be measured at this point with the markers on the catheter. The catheter should be inserted up to this point with the markers on the catheter. The catheter should be inserted up to this point when it is placed; for heavy individuals, 1 to 3 additional cm may be required to allow for the distance between the skin and the vein (Figure 3-2).

- Open catheter tray in sterile fashion and keep in easy reach.
- Uncap distal catheter lumen only, prepare the J-wire, draw 1% lidocaine into a syringe, and place 4 x 4-inch gauze pads in easy reach.
- Position needle snugly on syringe so that the bevel markings are opposite the syringe markings for easy viewing. The needle should be easy to remove so that it is not dislodged from the vein when the needle is removed after cannulation.
- Infiltrate skin at site of cannulation with 1% lidocaine using a 22-gauge needle. This needle may also be used as a "finder" needle for the vein itself. The needle should be inserted to the clavicle with lidocaine injected into the periosteum. Do not advance the needle unless the syringe is aspirated so that an arterial or venous puncture can be immediately detected.
- Keep the needle parallel to the floor and angled up toward the sternal notch, and lidocaine can be injected as the needle is slowly removed.
- Cannulate the vein at the clavicular angle (junction of the medial 1/3 and lateral 2/3). The skin will be penetrated very near the point where the vein is cannulated in thin or cachexic patients. In heavier individuals, the skin should be penetrated more inferior and slightly more lateral to allow an angle of attack to permit entry from under the clavicle into the vein (Figure 3-3).
- The cannulating needle should then be inserted through the anesthetized tract, contact should be made with the anesthetized portion of the clavicle, and the needle should be walked under the clavicle along the same path as the "finder" needle. Always aspirate the needle while advancing until venous blood is

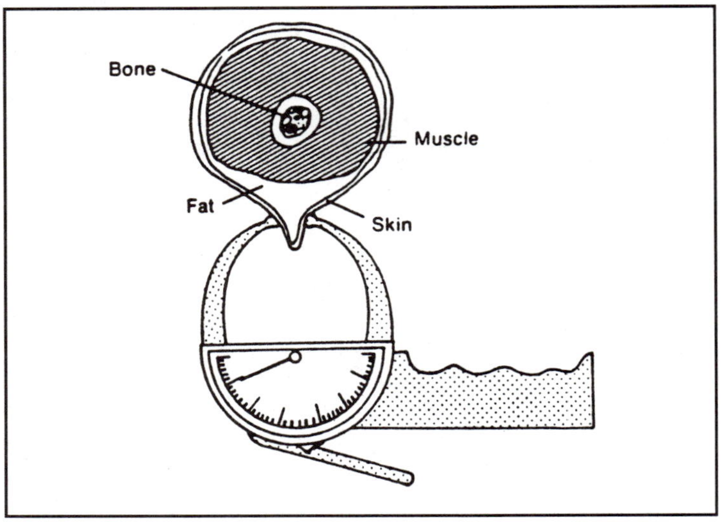

Figure 3-3. This cross-section shows the technique for measuring a skinfold, a double layer of subcutaneous fat and skin. In this case, the triceps skinfold is being measured with the Lang caliper. (Illustration from Grant, A. *Nutritional Assessment Guidelines*. Berkeley, California, Cutter Laboratories, 1979.)

returned. If no blood can be aspirated, the needle should be slowly withdrawn while aspirating because the vein may have been penetrated in a through-and-through manner. The lumen may be entered while withdrawing the needle.

- ✧ Stabilize the needle against the chest wall and remove the syringe once the vein has been cannulated.
- ✧ Advance the J-wire through the needle and into the vein.
- ✧ If resistance is encountered, withdraw the wire slowly and try again. If resistance to withdrawing the wire occurs, remove both wire and needle to avoid shearing off the end of the wire with the subsequent distal embolization.
- ✧ Withdraw the needle after half of the wire has been passed into the vein.
- ✧ Incise the skin at the site of entrance of the wire with a #11 blade (in kit) over the wire and into the vein. Twisting the dilator while advancing may help. Do not advance the wire with the dilator. Failure to pass the dilator may indicate a bent wire.
- ✧ Withdraw the dilator once it has been passed into the vein and apply pressure to the skin site to prevent bleeding.
- ✧ Insert the catheter over the guidewire until the wire emerges from the distal port. Grasp the wire and advance the catheter into the vein to the previously measured point.
- ✧ Remove the wire. Attach a syringe to the distal port to prevent venous air embolism.
- ✧ Flush the ports and fix the catheter to the skin with suture (Figure 3-4) and apply sterile dressing.
- ✧ Perform a chest radiograph to ascertain correct placement. If PN is being considered for a period of more than 2 weeks, a Hickman or similar cuffed, tunneled catheter is placed to reduce the risk of line sepsis. A percutaneously inserted central catheter (PICC) may also be appropriate.

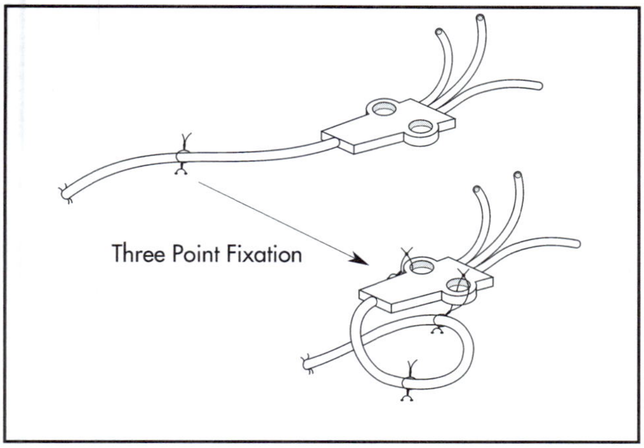

Figure 3-4. Flush the ports and fix the catheter close to the skin with suture. Illustration by Barbie Minnick.

Hickman, Broviac, or Groshong Catheter Placement

- Technique is the same as for a triple lumen catheter except that it is placed in the operating room where sterility is better controlled and additional sedation may be used if necessary.
- Two small skin incisions about 5 to 7 cm apart are necessary. The cuff should be placed just beneath the skin surface of the lower incision for easy removal under local anesthesia at a later date if necessary. The catheter should be well secured (Figure 3-5). It usually takes approximately 3 to 4 weeks for fibrous tissue to grow through the cuff. Therefore, the securing suture can be removed after that time if it is irritating for the patient.
- Proper tip placement in the vena cava should be verified by radiograph. A C-arm fluoroscope is unnecessary, costly, exposes the patient and personnel to additional radiation, and may be inferior to chest radiograph for determining proper catheter placement.

Catheter Care and Use Protocol

SITE CARE (ALL CATHETERS)

1. Clean catheter exit site with (3) alcohol saturated applicators, followed by (3) 2% chlorhexidine saturated applicators using the following principles:
   A. Apply in circular motion at site and work from center outward; do not reuse the same applicator over a previously cleaned area.
   B. Use single-use applicator, then discard; and use some type of applicator to avoid hand contamination.
2. Apply povidone-iodine ointment to the catheter exit site (optional).
   A. Dress with gauze or sterile transparent dressing. Gauze dressings should be changed daily or every other day; more often if saturated. Transparent dressings should be changed 1 to 3 times weekly. Dressings should be changed more frequently in neutropenic patients.

Figure 3-5. 4-0 purse-string to close. Illustration by Barbie Minnick.

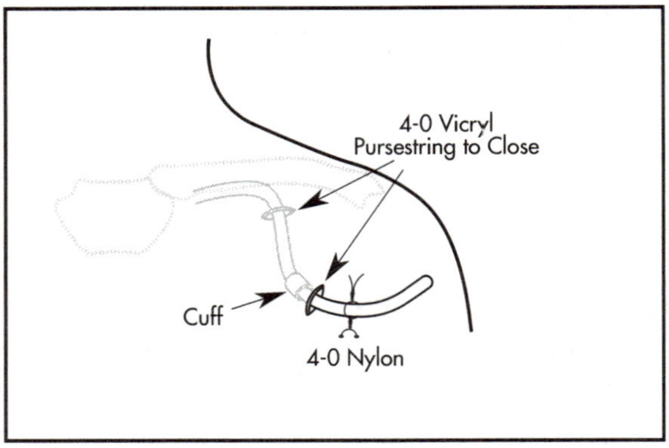

HUB CARE

Short-Term Central Venous Catheters (CVCs)	*Long-Term CVCs*
Scrub with chlorhexidine or povidone-iodine for 30 seconds prior to opening	Scrub junction with (3) alcohol Scrub junction with (3) 2% chlorhexidine or povidone-iodine Open port

The hub may be a common source for catheter infection.

CVC HUB CARE

CVC hub care should be done before any opening of the CVC at the level of the hub and prior to removal of CVC cap, cap change, tubing change, or tubing discontinuation.

Long-Term CVC Hub Care Procedure

(Tunneled silastic, PICC lines, subcutaneous infusion ports)

1. Clean work surface with alcohol and wash hands thoroughly.
2. Set up supplies
   (3) applicators saturated in 2% chlorhexidine or povidone-iodine
   (2) alcohol prep pads
   CVC occlusion forceps if no reattached clamps on line
   2-inch plastic tape
3. Use clean, non-sterile gloves if contact with blood or secretions is anticipated and remove tape at junction of the CVC hub and cap/IV tubing.
4. Scrub from catheter junction site outward in a circular manner—first using alcohol saturated applicators, then 2% chlorhexidine (or povidone-iodine) saturated applicators. Extend cleansed area approximately 2 inches on either side of the junction, then clamp CVC.
5. With alcohol prep wrapped around both sides of the junction, remove CVC cap or IV tubing. Continue to hold CVC with first alcohol wipe and perform necessary CVC care (cap change, tubing change, blood draw, heparin flush).
6. Replace CVC cap or IV tubing as necessary. Tape the junction securely with 2-inch plastic tape.

Short-Term CVC Hub Care Procedure

(Triple, double, single lumen, Cordis, Swan-Ganz, arterial lines)

Scrub hub with 2% chlorhexidine (or povidone-iodine) for 30 seconds. The latter must be permitted to dry prior to using CVC.

Injection Port Care

Scrub with 2% chlorhexidine (or povidone-iodine—must be permitted to dry prior to using CVC) 30 seconds before accessing port.

CVC Injection Port Care

CVC port care should be done before any entry of any injection port on the CVC or on IV lines connected to the CVC. This includes the following:

1. Injection cap ports.
2. Buretrol injection ports (not usually used with PN lines).
3. Injection ports on IV lines connected to CVCs.

Long-Term CVC Port Care Procedure

(Tunneled or short-term silastic, PICC lines, subcutaneous infusion ports)

Wash hands thoroughly. Use clean non-sterile gloves if contact with blood or secretions is anticipated, and scrub injection port vigorously with 2% chlorhexidine or povidone-iodine for 30 seconds.

IV Tubing Change

1. All IV tubing on all lines should be changed every 72 hours, except for TPN sets (amino acid/dextrose and intralipid solutions), which should be changed daily.
2. Portable computerized ambulatory drug delivery (CADD) (Deltec, St. Paul, Minn) and patient-controlled analgesic (PCA) units: tubing should be changed with cassette changes.
3. Stopcocks, y-connection, and extension sets should be changed with tubing changes.

CVC Care Principles

1. All procedures for CVC care are designed to prevent infections and mechanical complications of use. Aseptic technique should be maintained in all handling of the CVC and all attached lines.
2. Universal precautions should be observed at all times in handling the CVC.
3. For infusion in non-emergent situations after CVC placement, placement of catheter tip should be confirmed radiologically before it can be used for infusion.
4. The CVC multi-stick injection cap should be changed every week even if the catheter is not in use.
5. An infusion control device should always be used to administer primary IV fluids via the CVC to prevent blood backup and clot formation in the line.

CVC Dressing Care

The CVC exit site may be dressed with either:

1. Sterile gauze and tape—changed daily or every other day.
2. Sterile transparent dressing—change 1 to 3 times weekly.

The nurse may decide which type of dressing best meets the individual patient's needs. Patients who may not tolerate a sterile transparent dressing include:

1. Diaphoretic patients.
2. Patients with fragile skin (irradiated skin) or drainage at the CVC site.
3. Neutropenic patients.
4. Patient's preference should also be considered when dealing with patients with established CVCs.

Patients may develop irritation of the skin at the CVC site in response to the various cleansing agents used. Substitutions in cleaning agents may be made according to patient needs or preference.

Patients with Hickman, Broviac, or Groshong-type catheters that have been in place more than 2 to 3 weeks may shower or bathe. After a shower, the wet dressing is removed, skin is cleansed per protocol, and then redressed. If showering prior to this, the exit site and catheter should be covered with a watertight dressing.

CVC Dressing Change Procedure

1. Disinfect work area with alcohol and wash hands thoroughly.
2. Set up supplies:
   A. (3) applicators saturated in 2% chlorhexidine
   B. Povidone-iodine ointment (optional)
   C. Dressing—2 X 2 sterile gauze pad and tape or sterile transparent dressing
3. Have patient turn head away and remove old dressing. Look for erythema, drainage, or signs of catheter dislodgement at exit site.
4. Clean from exit site outward in circular motion, using the chlorhexidine-saturated applicators, cleansing an area of approximately 2 inches in diameter.
5. Apply small amount (pea-sized drop) of povidone-iodine ointment at exit site (controversial).
6. Apply dressing and secure the CVC to prevent dislodgement.

Percutaneously Inserted Central Catheters Line Dressing Guidelines

1. When removing old dressing, pull it off toward the shoulder to avoid dislodging catheter (in most cases, steri-strips will be used to secure the catheter in place). Alternatively, the PICC may be anchored to the skin using a suture. Cleansing may be done over/around the strips (if strips are intact). Strips must be changed weekly.
2. Newly placed PICC lines may require pressure dressing for the first 24 hours to prevent bleeding or hematoma formation. After this time, a transparent or gauze dressing should be placed. If insertion was difficult and the vein traumatized, a prophylactic heating pad used for 20 minutes every 6 hours over the next 24 hours may help prevent phlebitis.
3. The site may be covered with Kerlix (Kendall, Chicopee, Mass) if patient objects to the site of the PICC.

Heparin Flush Guidelines

Heparin flush is unnecessary for continuous infusions.

Heparin flush dosing: Standard heparin flush: 3 ml of 100 units/ml heparin (300 units) per lumen of CVC.

Pediatrics (and small adults): 50 units/kg body weight maximum per day (per day, not per flush or per lumen).

CVCs should be heparin flushed under the following circumstances:

1. When capped (not in use for continuous infusion): every 24 hours. (Exception: pediatric Arrow cath [Arrow, Reading, Pa], flush 4 to 6 hr when capped).
2. When discontinuing IV infusions, after administration of intermittent IV medications or fluids.
3. After CVC blood draws, as needed.

4. PICC Lines: 1.5 ml of 100 units/ml heparin (150 units).
5. Subcutaneous infusion ports: Standard heparin flush; 5 ml of 100 units/ml heparin (500 units) plus 5 ml of 0.9% sodium chloride. See Appendix A, Table 18—CVC care chart for other flushing guidelines.
6. Groshong CVC: Use 5 ml 0.9% sodium chloride for flushing. See Appendix A, Table 18—CVC care chart for other flushing guidelines.

Blood Drawing Via CVC

If coagulation studies are obtained through the CVC, it is necessary to aspirate 6 ml of blood before drawing samples for coagulation studies. Label requisition slip, "Drawn from _______ line."

The CVC may be used for drawing of blood cultures. The discard specimen may also be used for blood cultures.

Blood Drawing Via CVC Syringe Method

1. Determine amount of blood needed for tests ordered. Collect appropriate tubes and supplies; use clean, non-sterile gloves. Cleanse CVC hub using appropriate CVC hub care procedure and clamp all lumens of CVC. Lumens that are not being used for blood draw should remain clamped throughout procedure.
   Note: The following steps must be done quickly so the line does not clog.
2. Attach sterile syringe to CVC. Unclamp CVC and withdraw 6 ml of blood for discard unless the aspirated blood is to be returned, then clamp CVC and attach another sterile syringe.
3. Unclamp CVC and aspirate blood specimen. Continue steps 7 and 8 until all specimens are obtained, using a new sterile syringe each time. After appropriate specimens have been obtained, clamp CVC. The original aspirate may be returned at this time.
4. Flush CVC with 3 to 5 ml of 0.9% sodium chloride as necessary, followed by appropriate heparin flush. Recap the CVC or attach IV tubing to continue infusion and inject aspirated blood into appropriate tubes.

If needling through injection port to perform syringe blood draw:

1. Attach 20-gauge needles to blood draw syringes.
2. Cleanse injection port according to CVC injection port care procedure, before beginning procedure.

Vacutainer CVC Blood Draw Procedure

1. Determine amount of blood needed for tests. Collect appropriate tubes and supplies and a 7 ml red top blood collection tube for discard or clot for the blood bank if necessary.
2. Attach vacutainer and vacutainer Luer adaptor together (it is unnecessary to remove rubber cover of needle end inserted into vacutainer), and use clean, unsterile gloves.
3. Clean CVC hub using appropriate hub care procedure.
4. Stop infusion and clamp all lumens of CVC and disconnect IV tubing or cap on lumen to be used for blood draw.
5. Attach vacutainer to central line hub and unclamp CVC on blood draw lumen only and draw 7 ml for discard (use 7-ml red-top tube), then attach other blood specimen tubes to vacutainer to obtain ordered specimens (draw coagulation studies last). Clamp CVC after blood specimens are drawn and remove vacutainer.

6. Flush CVC with 3 to 5 ml of 0.9% sodium chloride as necessary, followed by appropriate heparin flush. Recap CVC or attach IV tubing to continue infusion.
7. Vacutainer holder is placed in plastic specimen cup containing alcohol (cover all of holder with alcohol).

If needling through injection cap to perform vacutainer blood draw:

1. Attach a 20-gauge needle, 1 inch long or less, into the Luer lock adaptor of the vacutainer holder.
2. Clean injection cap using CVC injection port care procedure.

Assessing Subcutaneous Infusion Ports

Subcutaneous infusion ports, or Port-a-caths (Deltec, St. Paul, Minn), may be accessed using a Huber needle for intermittent or continuous administration of IV fluids or medications.

1. Clean work surface with alcohol and wash hands thoroughly.
2. Assemble supplies:
   (3) applicators saturated with 2% chlorhexidine
   (1) pair sterile gloves
   (1) Huber needle ("Gripper" or standard)
      Gripper needle comes with extension set attached. If using standard Huber, attach microbore extension tubing to needle.
   (1) 5-ml syringe filled with 0.9% sodium chloride solution
3. Palpate port site to locate portal septum.
4. Clean area over port site with (3) 2% chlorhexidine-saturated applicators. With each applicator, start at the center of the port site and work outward in a circular motion to cover an area approximately 4 inches in diameter. Use sterile gloves.
5. Connect 5-ml syringe with sodium chloride to extension tubing on Huber needle and purge extension tubing and needle. *Maintaining sterility of the Huber needle is essential.*
6. Locate portal septum by palpation and insert Huber needle perpendicular to the septum, pushing it firmly through the skin and portal septum until it hits the bottom of the portal chamber.
7. Slowly inject approximately 3 ml of 0.9% sodium chloride into port, noting any resistance. Aspirate solution to check for blood return. If bubbling is observed around the needle when flushing, port may not be accessed properly. Remove needle and attempt to reassess port.
8. Slowly inject remainder of sodium chloride and clamp extension set and remove syringe, then attach appropriate IV tubing and administer solutions/medications as ordered.

Huber needle should be changed weekly when left in place for continuous infusion. Change dressing over port weekly.

Extension sets may be capped with multi-stick caps, and the port may be used for intermittent administration of IV fluids and medications. The port must be flushed daily and after each intermittent infusion under these circumstances. To remove Huber needle from port:

1. Clean work surfaces with alcohol and wash hands thoroughly.

2. Prepare supplies:
   A. 20-ml syringe filled with 5 ml of 100 units/ml heparin (500 units) and 5 ml 0.9% sodium chloride.
   B. Clean, non-sterile gloves.
3. Clamp extension tubing on Huber needle, clean junction, and disconnect IV tubing.
4. Attach 10-ml syringe with heparin and saline to extension tubing and unclamp extension tubing and slowly inject approximately 8 ml of heparin sodium chloride solution into port.
5. Withdraw Huber needle by maintaining positive pressure on syringe while simultaneously withdrawing the needle and pressing down on the port with 2 fingers. This will prevent reflux of blood into port.

Home Care

Patients requiring long-term central venous access may be discharged home with their CVC. It is not advisable to discharge patients with temporary-access CVCs such as percutaneous Cook (Bloomington, Ind) and Arrow catheters. All other types of CVCs may be considered safe for home use.

It is recommended that teaching for patients going home with a capped CVC begin at least 3 days before anticipated date of discharge. Ideally, patient teaching should begin as soon as it is known that the line will be placed. If the patient cannot care for the line, a family member or significant other should be identified to learn the necessary care procedures. *The patient and/or significant other should receive instruction in the following*:

1. CVC dressing change
2. Heparin flush of the CVC via injection cap
3. CVC injection cap change
4. Home problem-solving and follow-up care

It is helpful to provide the patient with written instructions accompanied by diagrams.

Components of Parenteral Nutrition Solutions

Fluid Volume

In a fluid-restricted patient, both dextrose and amino acid concentrations can be increased. A higher proportion of calories may also be supplied using lipid emulsion.

- The maximum glucose oxidation rate is 7 mg/kg/min.[7]
- For patients receiving continuous ambulatory peritoneal dialysis (CAPD), the amount of glucose absorption from the dialysate should be estimated and included in the calculation of delivered calories.

  Dialysis Solutions
  1.5% = 1.3 g/dL glucose
  2.5% = 2.2 g/L glucose
  4.25% = 3.76 g/L glucose

Absorbed glucose (g) = [11.3 (glucose conc. in dialysate) – 10.91 x volume of exchanges

Absorbed calories = glucose (g) x 3.7 kcal/kg

(Approximately 60% to 80% of glucose is absorbed)

Protein (Amino Acids)

Standard Formulations

Crystalline amino acids area available concentrations of 8.5% to 15%, although other concentrations can be provided for the proper indications. The amino acid solution is diluted with an appropriate amount of dextrose to achieve a desired concentration, usually 3.5% to 5.0%. These include a final concentration of <3.5% in non-oliguric renal and/or hepatic failure (in the absence of dialysis) or a final concentration of >4.25% in fluid restriction (see Appendix A, Tables 20 through 22 for protein supply and for the amino acid formulation of parenteral nutrition solutions).

Some amino acid formulas may contain sodium bisulfate as a preservative. Patients with hypersensitivity to sulfa should not receive these formulas.

Specialty Formulations

- High cost when compared with standard amino acid solutions.
- See Appendix A, Table 23 for the various specialty formulations available and their amino acid components.

Hepatic Disease (HepatAmine)

- High in branched chain amino acids.
- Low in aromatic amino acids.
- May be useful in patients with hepatic encephalopathy (grade II or greater or with chronic hepatic encephalopathy) who otherwise would be unable to tolerate sufficient standard amino acid infusion. If encephalopathy is secondary to sepsis, gastrointestinal hemorrhage, uremia, or electrolyte imbalance, there is no role for HepatAmine (Alpharma, Baltimore, Md). For further discussion, see *branched chain amino acids,* page 13.

Renal

See discussion on parenteral formulas.

High Branched Chain

See discussion on parenteral formulas.

Lipid Emulsion

- Lipid emulsions are isotonic and may be infused via peripheral vein. They are an especially valuable caloric source if peripheral parenteral nutrition is used.
- Used for a caloric source (typically 20% to 30% of total calories and to prevent essential fatty acid deficiency).
- 10% emulsion provides 1.1 kcal/ml and the 20% emulsion provides 2.0 kcal/ml (for comparison, D25 provides 0.85 kcal/ml and D35 1.1 kcal/ml) (see Appendix A, Tables 24 and 25 for caloric supply composition of lipid emulsions)
- A test dose of 0.5 ml/min over 15 to 30 min for 20% emulsion, or 1 ml/min for 10% emulsion is recommended to test emulsion stability and hypersensitivity.

- Maximum infusion rate is 100 ml/hr for the 10% emulsion and 50 ml/hr for the 20% emulsion to prevent overload of the reticular endothelial system.
- Maximum total infusion is 2.5 g/kg/day to avoid "fat overload syndrome" which is characterized by hepatomegaly, jaundice, thrombocytopenia, and death. Some evidence suggests <1.0g/kg/day may be associated with a lower incidence of liver disease.
- Maximum hang time for any bottle of lipid emulsion is 12 hours. There is evidence that 3:1 solution may be safely hung longer.
- Should not be used in patients who have allergy to eggs. Rare instances of anaphylaxis have been reported. Egg phosphatides are used as emulsifying agents.
- Uncommon side effects include fever, headache, back pain, dyspnea, chills, nausea, chest pain, and oily taste.
- May be used in pancreatitis not associated with hypertriglyceridemia as long as serum triglyceride concentration is monitored as with any other patient receiving intravenous lipids.
- No evidence in humans that the use of lipid emulsion induces premature labor.
- Soybean allergy is not a contraindication as the emulsion contains no soy protein.
- Triglyceride level should be checked 4 to 6 hours after the infusion has ceased to ascertain adequate clearance.
- Can be administered in a "piggyback" form with parenteral nutrition solutions via an injection port or administered directly. Lipid emulsion is also a constituent of 3 in 1 solutions (dextrose, lipid, amino acids).
- Lipids are not routinely administered through a filter unless 3 in 1 mixtures are used. In this situation, a 1.2-μm filter should be used to exclude particulate matter; bacteria will not be excluded. Filter pore size <1.2 μm will not permit lipid to pass.

Essential Fatty Acid Deficiency

Need minimum of 2% to 4% of total calories as linoleic acid for prevention (lipid emulsion is 50% linoleic acid).

Electrolytes

- Parenteral electrolyte content must be adjusted according to serum electrolyte concentration.
- Electrolyte imbalances should be corrected if possible before initiating PN.
- PN should not be used as replacement fluid for additional losses beyond maintenance.
- Sodium bicarbonate interferes with calcium-phosphate compatibility and should be avoided in parenteral nutrition solutions. Acetate salt should be used as a bicarbonate substitute. Sodium bicarbonate should never be injected through a catheter used for parenteral nutrition.
- To avoid alkalosis or hyperchloremic metabolic acidosis, the chloride to sodium ratio should be 1:1.

Acetate and Chloride

The pharmacist will balance the concentration of acetate and chloride in parenteral nutrition solutions to prevent hyperchloremic metabolic acidosis or hypochloremic metabolic alkalosis. In hyperchloremic metabolic acidosis, the acetate concentration can be maximized. This requires the addition of sodium and potassium (as acetate salts). The other option is to minimize the chloride concentration. This may be the only option if additional sodium and potassium cannot be added to the parenteral nutrition solution. Before manipulating the parenteral nutrition solution, attempt to correct any underlying disorder such as vomiting, diarrhea, or nasogastric suction losses.

PHOSPHATE

Phosphate is provided in parenteral nutrition solutions as either a sodium or a potassium salt. Therefore, when the phosphate concentration is increased from the standard, the sodium and/or potassium concentration should be correspondingly increased when possible. However, phosphate is ordered in mmol, not mEq, and is not in 1:1 ratio with the sodium or potassium salt (Tables 3-1 and 3-2).

CALCIUM-PHOSPHATE SOLUBILITY

The most commonly encountered compatibility problem encountered in parenteral nutrition solutions is the addition of calcium and phosphate. Precipitation may occur in the form of dibasic calcium phosphate crystals. These crystals may be apparent in the solution or become apparent only when the PN catheter lumen becomes occluded.

Calcium-phosphate solubility is dependent on several factors:

1. Relative molar Ca and P concentrations
2. Amino acid formula and concentration (the lower the concentration, the less soluble CaP)
3. Dextrose concentration (the lower the concentration, the less soluble CaP)
4. Temperature (less soluble at higher temperature)
5. pH of PN solution (dibasic precipitates form at high pH)
6. Order of compounding of the solution (Ca should be added last)

These variables make it difficult to set a maximum calcium or phosphate concentration. As a guideline, a maximum phosphate concentration of 17 mmol/L can be achieved with any solution containing calcium < 5 mEq/L. Phosphate concentration should never exceed 25 mmol/L even in solutions of high dextrose and amino acid concentration. Extraordinary Ca or P losses should be replaced separately from PN (Figure 3-6). Consult the pharmacy when additional Ca or P are necessary.

Vitamins and Minerals

- One vial of multivitamins should be provided daily in the first liter of parenteral nutrition solution.
- The vitamin concentrations in this formulation are based on the recommendations of the AMA Nutritional Advisory Group (see Appendix A, Table 26). Vitamin K is not a constituent of the multivitamin formulations.
- If the patient receives less than 1 liter of PN in a 24-hour period, the volume of vitamin and mineral infusion should be increased proportionately or one vial of multivitamins in 100 ml of D5W or 0.9% NaC1 should be administered over 2 hours.
- The multivitamin formula does not include vitamin K (phytonadione). However, 1 mg of vitamin K may be added daily to PN solution by the phar-

TABLE 3-1

Parenteral Phosphate Products

	Phosphate	Sodium	Potassium
Sodium phosphate	3mmol	4mEq	0
Potassium phosphate	3mmol	—	4.4 mEq

TABLE 3-2

Phosphate Conversion

Mmol PO4	ml added	mEq Na	mEq K
3	1.0	4	4.4
4	1.3	5	5.7
5	1.7	7	7.5
6	2.0	8	8.8
7	2.3	9	9.7
8	2.7	11	11.9
9	3.0	12	13.2
10	3.3	13	14.5

macy on a routine basis unless otherwise ordered. Therefore, the prothrombin time (PT) would not require weekly monitoring. Patients who are to be anticoagulated should not receive vitamin K.

✧ Long-term use of vitamin A should be avoided in renal failure because of the possibility of toxic accumulation as it is not removed during dialysis. Serum vitamin D and E levels should be monitored during renal failure (see Appendix A, Table 17 for information on signs of vitamin deficiency).

IRON

✧ Not routinely supplied in parenteral nutrition solutions, therefore, intravenous iron dextran (Imferon [Fisons, Crewe Crechshire, England] or iron gluconate) supplementation may be necessary. Iron dextran may not be available to the bone marrow.

✧ The dose may be calculated using the formula:

$$0.66 \times \text{body wt [kg]} \times \frac{(100 - \text{Hgb (g/dl} \times 100)}{14\text{g}}$$

For example, in an adult patient with a Hgb of 8.2 g/L weighing 68 kg:

$$\text{Iron deficit} = 0.66 \times 68 \times \frac{(100 - 8.2 \times 100)}{14.8} = 2925 \text{ mg}$$

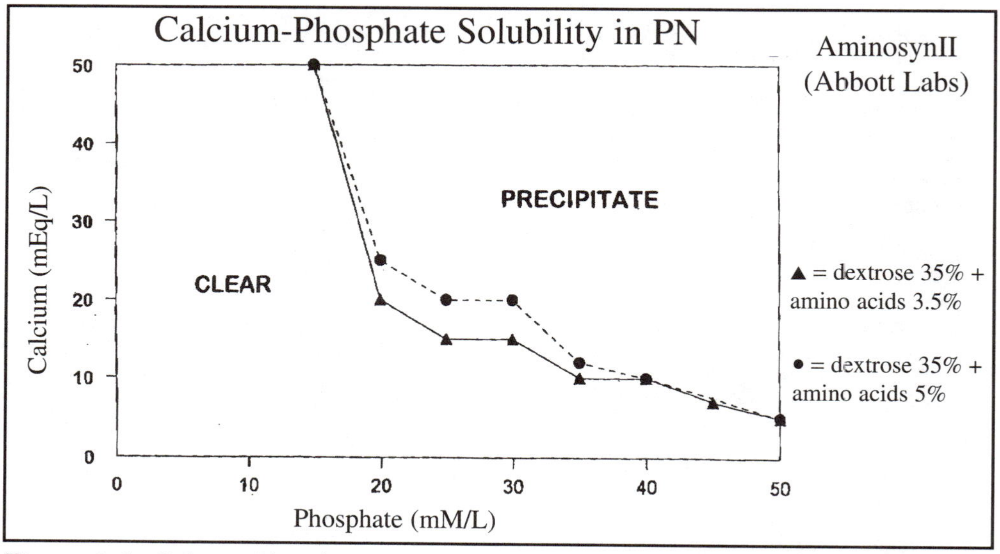

Figure 3-6. Calcium-Phosphate solubility in PN. Reprinted with permission from Abbott Labs, North Chicago, Ill.

Total amount of iron dextran necessary: Iron gluconate:

$$\frac{2925\text{ mg}}{50\text{ mg/ml}} = 58.5\text{ ml} \qquad \frac{2925\text{ mg}}{12.5\text{ mg/l}} = 234\text{ ml}$$

This may be infused in daily doses of 2 mL (100 mg—the maximum for 29 consecutive days in this case). The maximum dose is 100 mg daily because larger doses have been associated with severe arthralgias and paralysis (manufacturers' guidelines). Side effects have generally been associated with the dextron component and therefore it may be possible to give large doses of iron gluconate.

Before beginning iron dextran replacement, a free flowing IV is started and a "test dose" of 25 mg in 100 ml of 0.9 NaC1 is administered over 1 to 2 hours. The vein should be flushed with normal saline after the infusion is completed. Epinephrine (0.3 ml of 1:1000 solution) should be available at the bedside should anaphylaxis occur. Alternatively, iron dextran may be added to parenteral nutrition solutions, although the pharmacy should be contacted should non-standard additives be present in the solution because of limited compatibility data. No test dose is necessary with iron gluconate, but like iron dextron, it also is not compatible with TPN.

Trace Elements

One vial of multi-trace elements (zinc, chromium, manganese, copper, selenium) should be provided daily in the first liter of parenteral nutrition. Chromium and manganese supplementation may be unnecessary, but it is currently included in the multiple formulation.

- Copper and manganese should be withheld in cases of severe cholestasis.
- Selenium requirement may increase in renal failure.
- See Appendix A, Table 16 for signs of trace element deficiency.

- Sufficient iodine is supplied via povidone-iodine use and subsequent absorption through the skin.
- Nickel, molybdenum, vanadium, tin, silicon, fluoride, and arsenic may be required trace elements, but their necessity has only been demonstrated in animals.

Additives

Insulin

- If a patient's blood sugar is sufficiently elevated as to require a continuous insulin drip, PN should not be initiated until glucose is controlled. The blood glucose should be <200 mg/dL before PN is started.
- May be necessary to control glucose intolerance.
- When insulin is necessary, usually one unit of regular insulin per 10 g dextrose (eg, 10 units with D10, 25 units with D25) will be sufficient. This should be added directly to the parenteral nutrition solution during compounding. The suggested maximum insulin should be 2.0 units regular insulin per gram of dextrose (ie, 50 units/l of D25). If hyperglycemia continues, the dextrose concentration should be reduced and the source for the hyperglycemia investigated.
- A sliding scale should be ordered to cover hyperglycemic episodes despite the addition of insulin to the parenteral nutrition solution. However, the addition of a corresponding amount of insulin should be added to the parenteral nutrition solution of subsequently compounded bottles. No insulin or additional dextrose should be added to the bottle during the infusion as this violates the closed system and increases the risk of infection.
- If additional insulin is necessary, add 2/3 of the previous day's sliding scale dosage to the PN. Make certain to divide the total insulin dose by the number of liters of PN daily.
- The patient's glucose should be kept below 200 mg/dL to avoid glucosuria with subsequent fluid and electrolyte loss and during infections, impaired neutrophil chemotaxis and NK ability. However, because of the risk of overshooting and causing hypoglycemia, control below 120 to 140 mg/dL is undesirable except during pregnancy when the blood sugar should be <120 mg/dL.
- Insulin adsorbs to both glass and plastic bottles and tubing and this factor, though small, should be considered when determining insulin dosage, especially in highly sensitive diabetic patients.
- A sliding scale or *separate* continuous intravenous insulin infusion should always be used when insulin requirements are unstable to avoid the wastage of PN.
- Increased plasma insulin activates the NA-K ATPase pump, which shifts potassium intracellularly and decreases serum potassium concentration.

Heparin, Hydrocortisone

One thousand units of heparin and 5 to 10 mg hydrocortisone may be added to each liter of *peripheral* parenteral nutrition because evidence suggests a decrease in the risk of phlebitis.[2,8]

ALBUMIN

The use of albumin infusions in nutrition support is controversial. What is not controversial, however, is the fact that exogenous albumin infusion will not directly improve a patient's nutritional status. Albumin infusion, if used at all, should only be used specifically to improve plasma oncotic pressure and treat hypo-oncotic edema.[9] Albumin provides up to 75% of the normal oncotic pressure in the intravascular space especially when the serum concentration is <3.0 g/dL.[10] However, there is little increase in the oncotic pressure as the serum albumin increases above 3.0 g/dL.[11] It remains unclear if the provision of exogenous albumin leads to improved enteral formula tolerance in hypoalbuminemic patients. One study showed an improvement when serum albumin was increased from 3.0 to 3.4 g/dL[12] and another found that patients with a capillary oncotic pressure <18 mmHg had enteral feeding intolerance while those with a COP >18 mmHg did not.[13] Other studies have found that enteral feeding tolerance was unaffected by the serum albumin concentration and 97% of patients with an albumin <2.5 g/dL tolerated enteral feeding.[14,15] An area that has not been addressed in albumin infusion studies is the effect of albumin infusion on mitigating medication side effects due to alteration in drug delivery and elimination related to hypoalbuminemia.

If the use of albumin supplementation is contemplated, a slow infusion should be used rather than rapid bolus injection as the half-life is prolonged in the former and increased serum albumin concentration may persist for up to a week.[16] The total albumin deficit should be calculated and used as an endpoint in the use of supplemental albumin:

$$\text{Deficit (g)} = \text{weight (kg)} \times 3\ \text{dL/kg} \times 3.5 - \text{initial serum albumin g/dL}$$

The 3 dL/kg reflects the average percent of exchangeable albumin in the plasma compartment.[16]

H_2 ANTAGONISTS OR PROTEIN PUMP INHIBITION

H_2 antagonists may be added to parenteral nutrition solutions to control excessive gastric secretion in new onset short bowel syndrome, stress ulcer prophylaxis, or treatment of peptic ulcer disease. In fact, it is more cost-effective to add these medications to the parenteral nutrition solutions than to hang separate infusions. No currently available proton pump inhibitors are known to be stable in TPN and should therefore not be used in TPN solutions. If necessary, they must be infused separately. Oral H_2 antagonists as well as protein pump inhibitors are poorly absorbed in patients with intestinal failure.

ANTIBIOTICS

Typically, antibiotics are not added to parenteral nutrition solutions. However, consult Appendix A, Tables 28 and 29 for compatibility of the TPN line to be used for the antibiotic infusion. The use of a dedicated TPN line for additional infusions is discouraged if alternate infusion sites are available, unless catheter infection is being treated.

Writing Orders

Parenteral Nutrition Order Form

All orders for parenteral nutrition should be written on a parenteral nutrition order form so that all necessary ingredients can be easily ordered in their appropriate concentrations.

Orders to initiate TPN should contain indication, height, and weight. This is helpful for quality control and for basic nutritional assessment.

Any changes to the parenteral nutrition solution require the entire solution formula to be rewritten unless only the rate is changed. That way, the current PN formulation can be obtained from the patient record on an immediate basis if necessary, both in case of emergency and to save time by avoiding the need to search through the chart. If only the rate is changed, the Parenteral Nutrition Order Form should still be used, but only the new rate indicated and the form clearly marked "rate change only." (See sample Parenteral Nutrition Order Form, Figure 3-7.)

- Changes to the lipid emulsion order require the lipid emulsion section to be completely rewritten to limit the possibility of confusion.
- Make sure to indicate if currently infusing and previously ordered solution may be used before carrying out a new order (eg, "begin new order with next PN solution" or "may use previously mixed solution") to avoid waste. PN orders should be delivered to or faxed to the pharmacy as soon as possible to facilitate timely implementation. There is no such thing as an emergent requirement for TPN initiation.

Standard and Custom Solutions

Standard amino acid/electrolyte solutions have been developed to meet most patients' needs. These solutions will typically provide 1.0 to 1.5 g/kg/day of amino acids as well as maintenance quantities of electrolytes, minerals (except iron), and vitamins when administered in sufficient volume to meet the patient's maintenance fluid requirement. Caloric and protein intake can be adjusted by adjusting the PN infusion rate. Using standard solutions is cost effective and leads to fewer errors inherent in custom making each new solution. When a designated electrolyte, mineral, or trace element concentration is greater than the standard, more is added to the standard solution. However, when a lower quantity of an ingredient is ordered, the solution must be prepared from "scratch." PN solutions containing specialized amino acid formulas such as the branched-chain amino acid formulas may be substantially more expensive not only for the ingredient, but because the PN solution containing these ingredients must be made custom.

To avoid confusion when nonstandard solutions are necessary, write out the quantity for all electrolytes, minerals, vitamins, and trace elements so there is no confusion as to which concentrations are standard and which are not.

Initiating Parenteral Nutrition

Peripheral Parenteral Nutrition

A 60-kg patient (IBW 55 kg) is admitted with a partial small bowel obstruction. Indication: The patient is losing 1200 ml/day via NG suction and is NPO. Indication: except NPO >7 days due to small bowel obstruction.

Fluid Requirements

Maintenance: 1500 + 20 ml/kg > 20 kg		2200 ml
Replacement of NG losses:		1200 ml
	TOTAL	3400 ml

Protein Requirements

1 to 1.2 g/kg/day = 55 to 66 g/day

Caloric Requirements (Estimated)

33 kcal/kg/day (maintenance) (or preferably use direct calorimetry) = 1815 kcal

Suggested Regimen

1. 10% dextrose with 3.5% amino acid and standard electrolytes, minerals, vitamins, and trace elements at 100 ml/hr (2.4 l/day). This will provide 816 kcal and 84 g amino acids. Begin infusion at 100 ml/hr.
2. 20% lipid emulsion (500 ml) infused over 10 hours (50 ml/hr) with the parenteral nutrition solution to provide 1000 kcal/day. Serum triglyceride concentration should be checked 4 to 6 hours after the lipid infusion is completed to ascertain adequate clearance.
3. The appropriate replacement solution in this setting is 5% dextrose with 0.45% saline containing 20 mEq/L KCl infused at rate of ml/ml of NGT output (replaced every 8 hours).
4. Totals for proposed regimen:

   Calories: 1816 non-protein kcal (33 kcal/kg IBW)

   Amino acids: 84 g (1.5 g/kg IBW)

   (See sample Parenteral Nutrition Order Form, Figure 3-7 and Figure 3-8 on page 42.)

Note: In small patients, peripheral parenteral nutrition can provide complete nutritional requirements.

5. Maximize chloride and minimize acetate if patient is alkalotic.

Central (Total) Parenteral Nutrition

Example: A 55-kg patient (IBW 65 kg) is admitted with severe graft versus host disease (GVHD) with diarrhea and protein-losing enteropathy following a bone marrow transplant. A central line (Hickman catheter) is in place. Stool output is 8 liters daily.

Indication

GVHD and diarrhea

Fluid Requirements

Maintenance: 1500 ml + 20 mL/kg IBW		= 2400 mL
Replacement of diarrheal losses		= 8000 mL
	TOTAL	=10400 mL

Protein Requirements

1.5 g/kg/day = 98 g/day

Northwestern University Medical Center
676 N. St. Clair Street Chicago, IL 60611

Check Box:
☐ **Initiation Orders** ☐ **Change of Therapy** ☐ **Rate change only** ☐ **Discontinuation**
PN orders will not be filled by the pharmacy in the absence of indication and estimated needs unless rate change only. When change of therapy is checked, all PN solutions already made will be used unless otherwise ordered.

CONSULTS	Check Box: ☐ NST Clerk: Please notify
INDICATION FOR TPN	
ESTIMATED NEEDS	**Height** ____ inches **Current Weight** ____ kg **Ideal Body Weight** ____ kg Estimated caloric requirement ________ kcal/day (25-35 kcal/kg/day for maintenance, 40 kcal/kg/day for repletion) Estimated protein requirement ________ g/day (1.0-1.5 g/kg/day)* *May not be appropriate in hepatic or renal failure ☐ **Check box** to order **Indirect Calorimetry** to estimate resting energy expenditure and to determine caloric requirement.
FORMULA	**CHECK BOX FOR DESIRED FORMULA:**

1. PERIPHERAL **CENTRAL**
☐ Dextrose 10%-Amino Acid 3.5% ☐ Dextrose 25%-Amino Acid 4.25% ☐ OTHER ________________
(340 non-protein kcal/L) (35 g protein/L) (850 g/L non-protein kcal/L) (42.5 g protein/L)

2. ELECTROLYTES Check one:

☐ **Standard Electrolytes**		☐ **Custom Electrolytes** (Write as totals per L)		**Chloride and Acetate**
Na 35 mEq/L		Na ____ mEq/L		☐ Minimize Cl, max. Ac (for acidosis)
K 30 mEq/L	Mg 10 mEq/L	K ____ mEq/L	Mg ____ mEq/L	☐ Max. Cl, minimize Ac (for alkalosis)
Ca 5 mEq/L	P 10 mMol/L	Ca ____ mEq/L	P ____ mMol/L	☐ Balance CL & Ac
				☐ Ac ____ Cl ____

3. VITAMINS AND TRACE ELEMENTS
Unless otherwise ordered, MVI-12, Vitamin K_1 mg/day, and Multi-trace elements (Zn 3mg, Cr 12μg, Cu 1.2mg, Se 40μg, Mn 0.3mg) will be included in each daily TPN solution. Additional supplementation should be ordered under "Other".

4. ADDITIVES
Regular Human Insulin _____ U/L H_2 Blocker ____________ mg/24hrs Other ____________________

5. LIPID EMULSION Check Box
☐ 10% 500 ml (1.1 kcal/mL) ☐ 20% 200 ml (2.0 kcal/mL) ☐ 20% 500 ml (2.0 kcal/mL) Frequency_____

RATE	**Check one box and fill in blanks:** ☐ Start central PN at ___ mL/hr for ___ hrs, increase to ___ mL/hr for ____ hrs, then increase to ____ mL/hr thereafter (goal) ☐ Infuse at mL/hr **All fat emulsion infused at 50 mL/hr**
MONITORING	Nursing • Daily weights, strict inputs and outputs, temperature every 8 hours • Accucheck 2 hrs after every rate increase, then q.6h x 3 days (call M.D. if >200 mg/dL). Urine glucose BID • For discontinuation, PN rate to be decreased by 50% for 15 min. x2. Accucheck 30 and 60 min. after PN discontinued (central solutions only). Laboratory • Nutrition Panel I (electrolytes, BUN, creat., glu. Ca, Mg, PO_4) Day 1 & 2, then q.Mon. & Thr. • Nutrition Panel II (albumin, pre-albumin, total protein, LFTs) Day 1, then q.Monday • Triglyceride - Day 1 & 4, then q.Mon. (draw at least 4-6h after lipid infusion complete) • 24 hr urine for TUN (total urine nitrogen) on Day 4 & q.Mon

Time/Date Written: ____________________ Time/Date Noted: ____________________ Physician Signature: ____________________ Physician (Dictation) I.D. # ____________________	Addressograph

Figure 3-7. Adult parenteral nutrition solution orders.

Collect stool and urine for total nitrogen loss determination; requirement may be greater.

Caloric Requirements

Because the patient is 85% of IBW, this regimen should produce weight gain.

Rebuild tissue and weight gain: 40 kcal/kg/IBW = 2600 kcal/day

Suggested Regimen

1. 25% dextrose with 4.25% amino acids with standard electrolytes, minerals, vitamins, and trace elements (additional sodium, potassium, acetate, zinc, magnesium, and/or addition of selenium may be necessary depending on serum concentrations). Infusion at 100 ml/hr (2.41/day) will provide 2040 kcal and 102 g amino acids.
2. The solution should be infused at 40 ml/hr for 8 hr initially and glucose concentration (Accucheck [Roche Diagnostic, Basel, Switzerland]) determined after 2 hours. If the glucose is <200 ml/dl, the infusion rate should be increased by 25 ml/hr every 8 hours (with the glucose checked 2 hours after each rate increase) until the goal rate of 100 ml/hr is obtained.

3. 20% lipid emulsion (200 ml) infused over 6 hours to provide 400 kcal/day "piggybacked" with the TPN solution. The serum triglyceride concentration should be checked 4 to 6 hours after the lipid infusion is completed to ascertain adequate clearance. This is especially important in this case because cyclosporin may impair triglyceride clearance.
4. Maximize acetate and minimize chloride if patient is acidotic from diarrhea.
5. The appropriate replacement solution in this setting is 0.45% saline or normal saline containing 20 mEq/L KCI infused at a rate ml/ml of diarrheal losses every 8 hours.

Totals for Proposed Regimen
Calories = 2440 non-protein kcal (39 kcal/kg IBW)
Amino Acids = 102 g (1.6 g/kg IBW)
Fluid = 10 400 ml
(See Parenteral Nutrition Order Forms, Figures 3-7 and 3-8)

Monitoring of Parenteral Nutrition

Proper monitoring of patients receiving parenteral nutrition is essential to:

1. Detect and prevent complications.
2. Determine if proper and adequate nutritional ingredients are being infused.
3. Document positive clinical benefits.

The recommended laboratory tests and monitoring frequency are listed on the Parenteral Nutrition Order Forms (see Figures 3-7, 3-8). These include:

1. Initial measured weight and height; daily weights thereafter.
2. Temperature every 8 hours.
3. Strict input and output recording.
4. Blood glucose 2 hours after each rate increase for central PN and every 6 hours until patient is stable, then urine glucose each nursing shift thereafter.
5. Baseline blood tests (before PN):
   - Electrolytes, including Mg, Ca, P
   - Glucose
   - CBC with differential and quantitative platelets
   - Fe and TIBC and/or ferritin
   - PT
   - Total serum protein, albumin, prealbumin, BUN, and creatinine
   - Aspartate transaminase (AST), alanine transaminase (ALT), bilirubin, and alkaline phosphatase
   - Triglycerides
   - Zinc, chromium, selenium, or copper if clinically indicated
6. Tests performed daily until patient is stable (usually the first four days):
   - Electrolytes, including Mg, Ca, P
   - Glucose 2 hours after each rate increase and every 6 hours
   - BUN and creatitine
   - Triglycerides—once, unless elevated, 4 to 6 hours after lipid infusion completed

- ✧ When the patient is stable, these blood tests should not be repeated more than twice weekly, unless otherwise clinically indicated.

7. Laboratory tests performed weekly or biweekly:
   - ✧ AST, ALT, bilirubin
   - ✧ Total protein, albumin, prealbumin
   - ✧ Complete blood count (CBC) and platelets
   - ✧ Various trace elements if patient is receiving additional supplementation
   - ✧ 24-hour urine for TUN (or UUN if TUN is unavailable)

Patient Cost of Parenteral Nutrition

The cost of properly monitoring parenteral nutrition and of maintaining a central venous catheter should be considered when contemplating use of parenteral nutrition therapy. Patient charges for TPN and monitoring may be more than $1000 per day.

Complications of Parenteral Nutrition

Mechanical

Related to CVC Placement

- ✧ Pneumothorax
- ✧ Hydrothorax
- ✧ Catheter embolism
- ✧ Arterial puncture
- ✧ Air embolism—check tubing for air
- ✧ Central venous thrombosis
- ✧ SVC or inferior vena cava (IVC) syndrome
- ✧ Brachial plexus injury
- ✧ Myocardial perforation, cardiac tamponade
- ✧ Cardiac arrhythmias
- ✧ Catheter malposition
- ✧ Thoracic duct injury

Catheter Breakage

Silastic (Dow Corning, Midland, Mich) long-term CVC can be repaired if damage occurs along the external segment. Such catheters should be clamped only with smooth jawed plastic occlusion forceps; saw tooth clamps will damage the catheter.

When a silastic CVC is found to be damaged, the following steps should be undertaken immediately:

1. Clamp line with preattached CVC clamps or smooth jawed occlusion forceps between the patient and the damaged segment.
2. Disinfect area of damage with alcohol and povidone iodine and wrap with dry sterile gauze pad.

Northwestern University Medical Center
676 N. St. Clair Street Chicago, IL 60611

Check Box:
☒ **Initiation Orders** ☐ **Change of Therapy** ☐ **Rate change only** ☐ **Discontinuation**
PN orders will not be filled by the pharmacy in the absence of indication and estimated needs unless rate change only. When change of therapy is checked, all PN solutions already made will be used unless otherwise ordered.

CONSULTS	Check Box: ☒ NST Clerk: Please notify
INDICATION FOR TPN	Graft Versus Host Disease / Diarrhea
ESTIMATED NEEDS	Height 5'7" inches Current Weight 55 kg Ideal Body Weight 65 kg Estimated caloric requirement 2600 kcal/day (25-35 kcal/kg/day for maintenance, 40 kcal/kg/day for repletion) Estimated protein requirement 98 g/day (1.0-1.5 g/kg/day)* *May not be appropriate in hepatic or renal failure ☐ Check box to order **Indirect Calorimetry** to estimate resting energy expenditure and to determine caloric requirement.
FORMULA	**CHECK BOX FOR DESIRED FORMULA:**

1. PERIPHERAL
☐ Dextrose 10%-Amino Acid 3.5%
(340 non-protein kcal/L) (35 g protein/L)

CENTRAL
☒ Dextrose 25%-Amino Acid 4.25%
(850 g/L non-protein kcal/L) (42.5 g protein/L)

☐ OTHER ____________

2. ELECTROLYTES Check one:

☐ **Standard Electrolytes**
Na 35 mEq/L
K 30 mEq/L Mg 10 mEq/L
Ca 5 mEq/L P 10 mMol/L

☐ **Custom Electrolytes**
(Write as totals per L)
Na ____ mEq/L
K ____ mEq/L Mg ___ mEq/L
Ca ____ mEq/L P ___ mMol/L

Chloride and Acetate
☐ Minimize Cl, max. Ac (for acidosis)
☒ Max. Cl, minimize Ac (for alkalosis)
☐ Balance CL & Ac
☐ Ac ____ Cl ____

3. VITAMINS AND TRACE ELEMENTS
Unless otherwise ordered, MVI-12, Vitamin K_1 mg/day, and Multi-trace elements (Zn 3mg, Cr 12μg, Cu 1.2mg, Se 40μg, Mn 0.3mg) will be included in each daily TPN solution. Additional supplementation should be ordered under "Other".

4. ADDITIVES
Regular Human Insulin ∅ U/L H_2 Blocker Ranitidine 150 mg/24hrs Other ____________

5. LIPID EMULSION Check Box
☐ 10% 500 ml (1.1 kcal/mL) ☒ 20% 200 ml (2.0 kcal/mL) ☐ 20% 500 ml (2.0 kcal/mL) Frequency qD

RATE	**Check one box and fill in blanks:** ☒ Start central PN at 40 mL/hr for 8 hrs, increase to 70 mL/hr for 8 hrs, then increase to 100 mL/hr thereafter (goal) ☐ Infuse at ______ mL/hr **All fat emulsion infused at 50 mL/hr**
MONITORING	Nursing • Daily weights, strict inputs and outputs, temperature every 8 hours • Accucheck 2 hrs after every rate increase, then q.6h x 3 days (call M.D. if >200 mg/dL). Urine glucose BID • For discontinuation, PN rate to be decreased by 50% for 15 min. x2. Accucheck 30 and 60 min. after PN discontinued (central solutions only). Laboratory • Nutrition Panel I (electrolytes, BUN, creat., glu. Ca, Mg, PO_4) Day 1 & 2, then q.Mon. & Thr. • Nutrition Panel II (albumin, pre-albumin, total protein, LFTs) Day 1, then q.Monday • Triglyceride - Day 1 & 4, then q.Mon. (draw at least 4-6h after lipid infusion complete) • 24 hr urine for TUN (total urine nitrogen) on Day 4 & q.Mon

Time/Date Written: 8/28/95 1100 Time/Date Noted: ______ Physician Signature: [signature] Physician (Dictation) I.D. # 1234	Addressograph

Figure 3-8. Adult parenteral nutrition solution orders (completed).

3. Attempt to install a heparin flush as appropriate to protect patency of catheter while awaiting repair.
4. Order appropriate repair trays STAT from central supply: CVC specific repair kit (Hickman 1.6 mm repair kit), Hickman/Broviac repair tray.

CATHETER OCCLUSION (ALGORITHM 3-1)

The following may indicate catheter occlusion:

- Inability to infuse lipids even when dextrose/amino acid solution infuses
- Difficulty flushing the CVC
- Inability to withdraw blood from the CVC
- Blood back flow into the IV tubing

Catheter Thrombosis

- Treatment—Push administration of tissue plasminogen activator (TPA) or urokinase for clearing blocked CVCs.

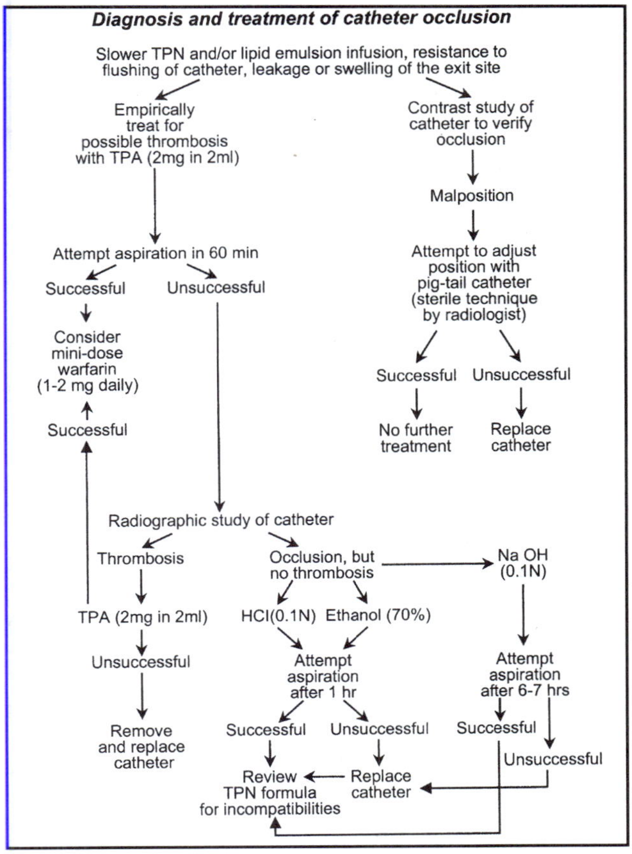

Algorithm 3-1. Diagnosis and treatment of catheter occlusion. (Reprinted from *Gastroenterology*, 124, 4, Buchman AL, et al, AGA technical review on short bowel syndrome and intestinal transplantation, 1111-1134, copyright 2003, with permission from the American Gastroenterological Association.)

- Rationale—Fibrin accumulation can cause partial or complete blockage of indwelling CVCs. Administration of a small volume of urokinase, a thrombolytic agent, IV push into the CVC may clear blockage of the internal lumen of the CVC without causing a systemic change in clotting times. Catheter occlusion may also result when the catheter becomes malpositioned either against the vessel wall or flips back into a smaller, more proximal vessel. If malposition is suspected, the catheter position should be assessed by radiology using radiopaque contrast.
- Contraindications (Allergy to urokinase or TPA)—If additional symptoms such as neck or face swelling, swelling of the limb proximal to the CVC or pain along the CVC tract with infusion exist, IV push TPA or urokinase should not be administered until a radiopaque dye study or ultrasound can be performed to rule out vascular thrombosis.
- Active internal bleeding, peptic ulcer disease, recent cerebrovascular injury, or intracranial/intraspinal surgery within the prior 2 months are contraindications for intravenous TPA infusion.

Procedure:

1. Lyophilized powder in vial (store in refrigerator).
   A. Draw up 2.2 ml of sterile water for injection (not bacterostatic).
   B. Allow bubbles to dissipate, then mix (without shaking) to dissolve (<3 min).

C. Use within 8 hours of reconstitution.

D. Inject appropriate volume into catheter or port.

E. Leave in catheter for 2 hrs. Then attempt aspiration of the catheter. If catheter is functional, flush with normal saline. If the catheter is not functional, repeat the procedure once.

Silastic CVCs (Hickman/Broviac-type CVCs)

Urokinase 5000 units/ml. Use 2 ml.

TPA 2 mg/ml. Use 2 ml.

Pediatric catheters/PICC lines (with extension tubing)

Urokinase 5000 units/ml. Use 0.6 ml.

TPA 2 mg/ml. Use 2 ml.

Instill 1 mg (2 mg if extension tubing)

Subcutaneous infusion ports

Instill 2 mg of TPA or 2500 units of urokinase.

Prevention of Recurrent Catheter Thrombosis

- ✧ In the absence of catheter malposition, patients are at increased risk for future catheter thrombosis and should therefore receive prophylaxis.
- ✧ Warfarin "mini-dose" (1 mg) or full anticoagulation with INR >1.6. Note that some patients with severe malabsorption may require increased doses of Warfarin; patients with residual colon incontinuity where vitamin K is synthesized may not.
- ✧ Lipid emulsion and multivitamin formulations contain vitamin K and may make larger Warfarin doses necessary.
- ✧ Low molecular weight heparin (30 mg SQ b.i.d.)

Non-Thrombotic Occlusion

Non-thrombotic catheter occlusions may be caused by poor solubility of Ca, P, and other divalent cations. Check PN formulation with pharmacy.

- ✧ If TPA or urokinase are unsuccessful in restoring catheter patency, non- thrombotic occlusion should be considered. Hydrochloric acid (HCl) may be used in clearing mineral precipitate.[17]
- ✧ 0.2 to 0.5 ml of sterile 0.1 NHCl is instilled using a 1-ml syringe. Re-prep catheter up. Wait 20 minutes and attempt to aspirate. This may be repeated 2 more times if necessary. Leave HCl in the catheter for 1 to 3 hours before attempting to re-aspirate. If successful, flush the catheter with 3 to 5 ml of 0.9% sodium chloride followed by a heparin flush.

Infections

See Algorithm 3-2.

Central catheters become infected at 3 sites: skin entry site, the catheter hub, and the fibrin sheath coating the outside of catheter inside the vein.

Catheter Sepsis

This is the greatest concern in patients receiving parenteral nutrition because an indwelling catheter is a potential conduit for organism entry from skin contamination, and a malnourished or debilitated patient may be immunocompromised and,

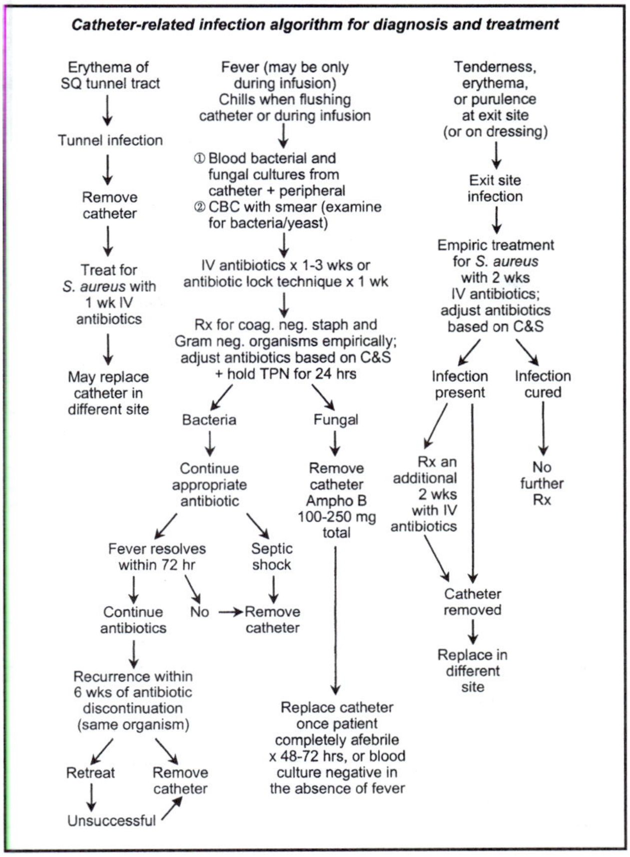

Algorithm 3-2. Catheter-related infection algorithm for diagnosis and treatment. (Reprinted from *Gastroenterology*, 124, 4, Buchman AL, et al, AGA technical review on short bowel syndrome and intestinal transplantation, 1111-1134, copyright 2003, with permission from the American Gastroenterological Association.)

therefore, is a good host for infection. Using aseptic and following prescribed catheter care protocols are essential for minimizing infections.

Evaluation of Fever

- If any fever greater than 38.5°C develops during the administration of parenteral nutrition, close examination for a focal source must be undertaken. Fever may also be associated with allergic reactions to the nutrients (rare), other drugs, or contaminated solutions (rare).
- Blood cultures for bacteria and fungi should be obtained both from the catheter and peripheral vein. Sterile techniques is particularly important. Also check CBC with differential, urine, and chest radiograph.
- Antibiotics should usually be withheld unless it is clinically obvious the patient has a catheter infection (eg, rigors after flushing catheter), the patient continues to spike a fever for more than 8 hours, or the patient progresses to septic shock. The PN nutrition solution should be held, but alternative electrolyte solutions should still be administered if necessary through a new catheter. If the patient defervesces with holding the nutrient solution and re-spikes a fever with continuation of parenteral nutrition, that suggests either the catheter or the solution is the source. Samples of the nutrient solution should be sent for culture. Remember that sepsis can occur in the absence of fever or leukocytosis. If the catheter is a temporary (non-Hickman, "Broviac") type, it should be removed, the tip should be sent for culture, and broad spectrum aerobic gram positive and negative antibiotic coverage should be initiated.

Vancomycin and an aminoglycoside or third generation cephalosporin are started as empiric coverage to cover for *Staphylococcus epidermidis, S. aureus,* and *E. coli,* the most common infecting organisms. *Pseudomonas* is not commonly an infecting organism. Patients receiving parenteral nutrition may occasionally be infected with unusual organisms, and these should not necessarily be dismissed as contaminants. Quantitative blood cultures obtained from the catheter may be useful.

- Antibiotic therapy can be tailored to an individual organism once a positive identification and sensitivity are available. Fastidious gram negative organisms may require up to 4 days for growth to be detected in culture media. Because of the potential toxicity of anti-fungal therapy, no empiric use of amphotericin is indicated unless yeast are detected on the peripheral blood smear. If catheter-associated sepsis is documented, the catheter should be removed if it is a temporary catheter and antibiotics infused for 7 days. Fungal infections require 250 to 500 mg of amphotericin over the total course of therapy. Caspofungin may also be used. The loading dose is 70 mg IV, followed by 50 mg daily for 14 to 28 days. A new catheter can be placed and parenteral nutrition resumed once the patient has been afebrile on antibiotics at least 48 hours.
- Every attempt should be made to preserve Hickman and Broviac type catheters. Catheter-associated sepsis can often be treated successfully by leaving the catheter in-situ.[18] That is especially important for a patient requiring permanent TPN who may have few sites for venous access. However, antibiotics must be infused for 14 to 28 days. If the patient remains febrile 72 hours after antibiotic therapy is initiated or develops progression of the sepsis syndrome, (including but not limited to renal, respiratory, or cardiac failure, disseminated intravascular coagulation [DIC], endocarditis, or embolism), the catheter should be removed immediately. The catheter must always be removed in the event of a systemic fungal infection. For patients requiring home TPN, antibiotics can also be infused at home although only daily to twice daily regimens are feasible. The patient can be trained by the nursing staff/nutrition support nurse and home health nurses to do this.

Exit and Tunnel Site Infections

These infections usually occur in the absence of fever or leukocytosis. They are identified by local tenderness, purulent exudate and/or erythema at the catheter exit site. Temporarily catheters should be removed and the exudate cultured. The usual organisms are *S. aureus* or *S. epidermidis* and intravenous vancomycin should be initiated pending culture results. Antibiotics should be continued for 5 to 7 days even in the absence of positive cultures. In the event of an infected Hickman or Broviac type catheter, an attempt should be made to treat the catheter in-situ with intravenous vancomycin. One to 2 weeks of antibiotic therapy are usually necessary, and the success rate is approximately 50%. Care should be taken to exclude a *tunnel infection.* This is an infection of the subcutaneous tunnel that the catheter follows under the skin. This infection cannot be treated without catheter removal. It is indicated by a red streak and tenderness of the skin overlying the tunnel tract.

Metabolic Complications

Hyperglycemia

If a patient spills 2+ or greater glucose in the urine on 2 or more consecutive occasions or blood glucose is ≥200 mg/dL:

- The usual initiation rate should be approximately 2 to 3 mg/kg/min of dextrose (ie, 40 ml/hr for D25).
- Consider drug interactions with the test system.
- Verify the infusion rate and ensure that no "catching up" has been attempted in the event the patient may have missed a portion of his daily parenteral nutrition.
- Check serum potassium. Glucosuria may be secondary to hypokalemia, and this can be corrected without insulin administration.
- Check for sepsis or other infections. Hyperglycemia may often occur prior to fever. Chromium deficiency has been poorly documented in humans and has been only *possibly* described in 3 case reports. Therefore, it is extremely unlikely that chromium deficiency would account for the hyperglycemia.
- Should it be necessary to add insulin, initially add 1 unit per 10g dextrose (eg, 10 units for D10W). Orders should be written to cover the patient with sliding scale insulin dosing in the event that 1 unit per 10 dextrose is insufficient. Additional insulin can be added to the *next* TPN bottle. It is inappropriate to regulate the patients serum glucose below 150 mg/dL unless symptomic from glucosuria. Finer control is rarely possible and places the patient at risk for hypoglycemia. If hyperglycemia persists despite the use of >2.0 units insulin per g dextrose, the level of dextrose infusion should be decreased. An attempt should be made to gradually decrease the insulin dose once blood glucose concentrations are consistently ≤120 mg/dL.
- The daily urine volume can be multiplied by the energy value glucose (3.75 kcal/g) to estimate the energy loss from glucosuria.

Hypoglycemia

- Hypoglycemia may occur with abrupt cessation of central PN. Therefore, concentrated dextrose infusions (>10%) should be tapered before cessation.
- Tapering may be performed by decreasing the PN rate by 50% for 15 minutes, and then another 50% for 15 minutes, then disconnect. For the rare patients who develop hypoglycemia after this tapering, future taperings can be extended to 45 to 60 minutes. It is for this reason the blood glucose should be checked 30 and 60 minutes after TPN after TPN with a <10% dextrose concentration is discontinued.
- In a "Code Blue" situation, PN should be immediately discontinued and 10% dextrose simultaneously substituted.
- Hypoglycemia may occasionally be the initial manifestation of sepsis even in the absence of fever or leukocytosis.

Electrolyte Imbalances

- The most common electrolyte imbalances are related to potassium, phosphorus, and magnesium. Abnormalities in serum calcium occur less frequently.

During protein synthesis, the serum concentration of these ions may decrease (see re-feeding syndrome).

- Hyperchloremic metabolic acidosis may be treated by the substitution of acetate for the chloride salts of Na and K. The underlying cause of metabolic acidosis or alkalosis should be corrected before manipulating the parenteral nutrition solutions. Bicarbonate itself may not be added to parenteral nutrition solutions due to imcompatibilities. Abnormalities in serum calcium occur less frequently.
- The tendency to "chase" slight variations in lab tests with frequent changes in the electrolyte content of parenteral nutrition solutions is to be avoided because this is expensive and leads to waste. Whenever possible, deficiencies should be corrected with separate "piggybacked" bolus infusions. Stable, increased electrolyte requirements may be met by addition to the parenteral nutrition solution. Sources of electrolyte loss such as nasogastric suction, diarrhea, or fistula drainage should be identified and replaced separately from PN. Most important, iatrogenic electrolyte abnormalities can be minimized by appropriate monitoring, especially when the PN solution is changed.

Elevated BUN

Elevated BUN may be caused by either catabolism due to insufficient calories and/or protein, or excessive protein intake. The differential diagnosis should also include dehydration, renal insufficiency, and gastrointestinal hemorrhage. Drug therapy should be re-evaluated in situations where an elevated BUN is encountered.

Hepatic Aminotransferase Elevation

Elevation of ALT, AST, and/or alkaline phosphatase may occur 2 to 14 days after initiating parenteral nutrition. The ALT and AST return to normal or near normal without disconnecting the parenteral nutrition. Alkaline phosphatase may remain mildly elevated due to the cholestatic effects of parenteral nutrition, biliary sludge (which occurs in 100% of patients receiving parenteral nutrition in the complete absence of oral intake after 4 weeks), a calculous cholecystitis, or metabolic bone disease. A normal or low alkaline phosphatase may be associated with zinc deficiency.

Elevation of ALT and/or AST may be related to overfeeding, excessive dextrose infusion, insufficient lipid infusion, excessive lipid infusion, choline deficiency, medications, or pre-existing liver disease such as chronic hepatitis. Choline supplementation is currently available for investigational use only. The bilirubin is seldom elevated in adults. Over the short term, liver test abnormalities are usually without consequence although right upper quadrant pain secondary to hepatic steatosis-induced hepatomegaly may occur. Chronic liver disease and hepatic failure secondary to parenteral nutrition, while common in neonates, is uncommon in adults until the patient has received several years of parenteral nutrition.

Cholecystitis

Calculous cholecystitis or acalculous cholecystitis may occur in up to 40% of patients receiving long-term parenteral nutrition. Gallstones may be either cholesterol or pigmented stones, and there is a relationship with decreased gallbladder motility and decreased cholecystokinin CCK release; 100% of patients receiving TPN will form biliary sludge after 4 weeks. It is therefore important to encourage some oral intake if at all possible. The use of parenteral CCK is expensive and occasionally associated with nausea, vomiting, and abdominal pain and therefore is not routinely recommended.

Gastroparesis

Both dextrose/amino acid solutions and lipid emulsions have been associated with delayed gastric emptying and perhaps early satiety. This effect may persist for some period even after TPN is discontinued.

Lipoprotein Abnormalities

An elevation in serum triglycerides may be seen because of the lipid infusion. Serum concentrations >250 mg/dL may lead to impairment of the reticular endothelial system. Impaired triglyceride clearance may occur in renal failure or with the use of cyclosporin; it does not occur during cirrhosis. Serum triglycerides 1000 mg/dL may cause pancreatitis and should definitely be avoided. The rate and total infusion of lipid emulsion should be reduced as necessary although a minimum of 2% to 4% of total calories as linoleic acid must be provided to prevent essential fatty acid deficiency. Serum triglycerides should be measured 4 to 6 hours after lipid infusion has been completed. If an elevated concentration is found, the phlebotomy time should be determined to ascertain if it occurred *during* the lipid infusion. In contrast to triglycerides, hypocholesterolemia often occurs during TPN, although both low-density lipoproteins (LDLs) and high-density lipoproteins (HDLs) are equally affected. No known abnormalities related to this have been described although the effects on wound healing are unknown.

Metabolic Bone Disease

Osteopenia is a characteristic of patients receiving long-term PN. It is a heterogenous disease and may include either osteoporosis or osteomalacia and may be associated with bone pain. A correlation with serum fluoride concentration has been identified in humans but fluoride supplementation is currently not approved or recommended. Aluminum contamination of parenteral nutrition solutions was a problem before 1986. Some patients receiving parenteral nutrition may have elevated parathyroid hormone (PTH) with resultant osteoporosis, probably because of insufficient Ca infusion or renal insufficiency although others have normal or suppressed PTH. The etiology of metabolic bone disease during parenteral nutrition is the subject of ongoing investigation.

Renal Insufficiency

Decreased glomerular filtrate rate has been observed in patients receiving long-term parenteral nutrition. The etiology may be partly related to excessive chromium infusion and systemic infections, but is mostly undefined.[19]

Refeeding Syndrome

If nutritional repletion is over-vigorous or achieved too rapidly in severely malnourished patients, refeeding syndrome may result. The serum phosphate concentration may decrease dramatically because of the intracellular movement of the ion for ATP production. The result can be hemolysis, cardiac dysfunction, neuromuscular dysfunction including sensory loss, paralysis, seizures, rhabdomyolysis, and respiratory failure.[20] Serum K and Mg may also decrease abruptly because of intracellular shifts. Therefore, nutritional repletion, especially with carbohydrate energy sources, should proceed gingerly over the first week with serum P, K, and Mg determined daily. There may be additional safety value in using a high protein formula for repletion at this time.

Initiating nutritional therapy too rapidly may also lead to fluid overload, increased metabolic rate, and subsequent congestive heart failure. The body adapts to starvation by lowering resting energy expenditure. If the patient is well below IBW, use *actual* body weight to calculate initial nutritional requirements and set reasonable caloric goals (ie, 30 to 35 kcal/kg/day). It may be wise to begin parenteral as well as enteral nutrition therapy with as little as 20 kcal/kg/day IBW in a severely malnourished patient. Indirect calorimetry should be performed if possible on all severely malnourished patients because estimates of caloric requirements in this setting may have a significant degree of inaccuracy, and miscalculation can lead to undesirable patient outcome in this group. It is prudent to initially restrict dextrose calories to reflect endogenous glucose synthetic rate (2 mg/kg/min or 150 to 200 g/day) to avoid hyperglycemia and hyperinsulinemia, the latter of which will lead to further decreases in serum potassium concentration. The increased serum insulin also promotes an antidiuretic effect, which can lead to fluid overload and further cardiac decompensation. The level of protein repletion does not need to be decreased.

Overfeeding

The provision of more than 40 kcal/kg IBW/day will not accelerate protein and tissue synthesis. Overfeeding can cause significant metabolic complications including hepatic steatosis, hyperglycemia, and excessive CO_2 production. The latter may precipitate respiratory failure or inhibit successful ventilator weaning in patients with marginal respiratory reserve. Severe and potentially life-threatening hypophosphatemia, hypokalemia, and/or hypomagnesemia may also develop.

Intestinal Morphology and Functional Changes

Frank intestinal atrophy associated with the use of TPN and lack of oral enteral intake has not been demonstrated in humans. TPN is associated with a decrease in villus height and an increase in intestinal permeability in humans. However, the clinical significance of this finding is currently undefined in humans.

Home TPN

Assessment and Training

- Requires proper training of the patient or significant other in proper catheter care techniques, use of an IV pump, preparation of TPN solutions for infusion, and IV antibiotic use (if necessary). Do not discharge the patient home until he or she has demonstrated safety and proficiency in their personal care.
- Family members can often be trained to prepare the solutions and to connect and disconnect the TPN. Alternatively, a social worker may be successful in finding a suitable trainee but is often unsuccessful, and this will involve additional, often unreimbursed expenditures.
- The capability of the patient for family for home TPN should be properly assessed before referral. This includes:

  - Patient or significant other manual dexterity, aptitude, and compliance
  - Home environment including location, site of solution preparation, overall cleanliness, and designated extra refrigerator
  - Indication for home TPN including progression or prognosis of the underlying disease
- Requires the patient to be metabolically stable without requiring frequent adjustment in their TPN prior to hospital discharge.
- Early referral of potential home TPN patients allows for a smoother transition. For example, patients with endstage cancer who are bedridden expected to live only 1 to 2 months may not be appropriate candidates.
- Family or significant other support.
- Finances. Home TPN can be extraordinarily expensive (well over $100,000 per year). Alternative financial sources may require early exploration.

Preparation for Discharge

- The hours of TPN infusion should be "cycled" or compressed into a night time infusion schedule prior to discharge (Cycling TPN Order Form, Figure 3-9). This permits the patient to perform usual activity during the day (including gainful employment) and to receive TPN overnight while asleep. See TPN cycling schedule (Table 3-3).
- A 10- to 12-hour infusion cycle is usually the goal. The infusion period is compressed while the total infusion volume remains unchanged. Some patients may require a slower infusion rate and longer infusion time because of the inability to tolerate the fluid load.
- The blood glucose (Accucheck is acceptable) should be checked 2 hours into each infusion period that the rate is increased. The addition of regular insulin to the PN solution is sometimes necessary. Insulin should not be added to the PN solution once it is already infusing.
- To taper TPN, reduce the rate by 50% for 15 minutes, and then by another 50% for another 15 minutes before it is discontinued. The taper period may be extended to 45 to 60 minutes with smaller incremental rate reductions for patients who develop hypoglycemia with the standard taper.
- Tapering is not included in the infusion time.
- Blood glucose should also be checked 30 and 60 minutes after the PN is tapered off because the high concentration dextrose infusion (at rapid rate especially) stimulates insulin secretion and may result in "reactive" hypoglycemia. The body "adapts" to this phenomenon on a more chronic basis, and once the blood glucose is acceptable after the tapering, home monitoring is seldom necessary unless the patient develops symptoms of hypoglycemia. It may also be necessary to decrease the dextrose concentration if the blood glucose cannot be satisfactorily controlled. Patients can be taught to add insulin to the TPN solution, but this should only be done when preparing the solution only (prior to hanging the bag).
- The PN solution at home consists of a single 2- to 3-liter bag, which may differ from that used in the hospital. Three-in-one bags, in which the lipid emulsion is combined with the dextrose/amino acid formula are becoming increasingly popular. However, the patient or significant other must carefully inspect the

Northwestern University Hospital 676 North St. Clair Street, Chicago, IL 60611
Use Ball Point Pen—Press Firmly

CYCLING: The process of changing the TPN regimen from a continuous infusion t a shortened, fixed infusion. It is generally suggested to compress the total 24h volume of TPN by 2h increments for each subsequent 24h period.

WEANING OFF TPN: Decrease infusion rate by half for 15 minutes; again decrease infusion rate by half for 15 minutes; stop TPN, flush and cap lumen. Fat infusion to run over same time duration as TPN.

Cycling orders as follows:

Present TPN is infused @ ______ ml/Hr over 24 hours QD providing __________ml/day

Day 1: Beginning __________, __________start compression
(Date) (Day)

Discontinue TPN __________
(Time)

RESTART TPN @__________, @__________ml/h
(Time) (Rate)

Day 2: On __________, COMPRESS TPN @ __________
(Date) (Time)

RESTART TPN @__________, @ __________ml/h
(Time) (Rate)

Day 3: On __________, COMPRESS TPN @ __________
(Date) (Time)

RESTART TPN @__________, @ __________ml/h
(Time) (Rate)

Day 4: On __________, COMPRESS TPN @ __________
(Date) (Time)

RESTART TPN @__________, @ __________ml/h
(Time) (Rate)

Day 5: On __________, COMPRESS TPN @ __________
(Date) (Time)

RESTART TPN @__________, @ __________ml/h
(Time) (Rate)

Day 6: On __________, COMPRESS TPN @ __________
(Date) (Time)

RESTART TPN @__________, @ __________ml/h
(Time) (Rate)

Day 7: On __________, COMPRESS TPN @ __________
(Date) (Time)

RESTART TPN @__________, @ __________ml/h
(Time) (Rate)

After desired rate is achieved, continue cycling schedule as ordered on day __________.

Once each day, after stopping the TPN, flush each lumen of the central line with HEPARIN 100 units. Chart time and number of lumens on the MAR.

OBTAIN ACCUCHECK ______ hours and ______hours after restarting TPN for ______ days. Also obtain accuchecks 30 min. and one hour after the end of infusion.

OTHER INSTRUCTIONS

Time/Date written: ____________________ Addressograph:

Time/Date noted: ____________________

Physician Signature: ____________________

Physician (Dictation) I.D.#: ____________________

Figure 3-9. TPN cycling orders.

Table 3-3

TPN Compression Schedule

	1 liter/night		2 liters/night		3 liters/night	
Day	**Rate**	**Hours**	**Rate**	**Hours**	**Rate**	**Hours**
1	42 ml/hr	24	83 ml/hr	24	125 ml/hr	24
2	45	22	90	22	136	22
3	50	20	100	20	150	20
4	55	18	111	18	166	18
5	62	16	125	16	187	16
6	71	14	142	14	214	14
7	83	12	166	12	250	12
8	100	10	200	10	300	10

bag for cracking or creaming of the emulsion prior to use. Alternatively, the lipid emulsion may be "piggybacked" into the TPN line.

- The solution comes premixed from the pharmacy. However, the patient or significant other must add the vitamin preparation immediately before use because some vitamins may destabilize especially if exposed to light over time. The patient or significant other can be taught to add other additives including H_2 blockers or insulin if necessary. The number of additives that the patient is required to add in the home environment should be minimized. It is wise to use as few additives as possible. Each additional entry into the bag creates additional work and inconvenience, and worse, may increase the risk of poor technique and increase the risk of infection.
- Daily TPN and/or infusion may not be required for some patients who may have sufficient absorption to allow for partial TPN support (eg, 3 to 6 times weekly).

Complications

- There is a significant risk of biliary sludge formation and the development of gallstones associated with long-term TPN. Therefore, patients should be allowed and encouraged to eat some if possible, even if their absorption is negligible. Most patients will prefer to eat simply for the pleasure involved, but oral food intake will help stimulate gallbladder contractivity and prevent sludge formation. Some oral intake may also be advisable to prevent intestinal complications associated with TPN although the clinical significance of this is yet unclear.
- Patients or significant others should be instructed that the first sign of catheter occlusion may be the inability to infuse the lipid emulsion. They should contact their physician if difficulty with the TPN infusion is encountered.
- Patients or significant others should be instructed that the first manifestation of sepsis may occur when chills are encountered while hooking up or flushing

the catheter after disconnection. They should immediately contact their physician. Patients should also check the catheter site daily for redness or purulent drainage.

- If fever develops during the TPN infusion, the patient or significant other should be instructed to taper the TPN off in the usual manner, contact the physician who should be familiar with infections associated with central venous catheters and the treatment, and report immediately to the emergency room or clinic.
- Patients may occasionally experience muscle cramping during the TPN infusion. This may be due to intra- and extravascular electrolyte shifts and is usually alleviated by decreasing the infusion rate. This will require a longer infusion period.
- Dehydration can occur with TPN if hyperglycemia develops or appropriate additional replacement fluids are not infused. Patients with short gut syndrome, chronic diarrhea, or high output fistuals, for instance, may require additional replacement fluid, which can usually be infused simultaneously with the TPN—either as part of the TPN bag or separately in a "piggy-backed" manner. This requires additional patient or significant other instruction.

References

1. Makarewicz PA, Freeman JB, Fairfull-Smith R. Prevention of superficial phlebitis during peripheral parenteral nutrition. *Am J Surg.* 1986;151:126.
2. Tishe MS, Wong C, Martin IG, et al. Do heparin, hydrocortisone, and glyceryl trinitrate influence thrombophlebitis during full intravenous nutrition via a peripheral vein? *JPEN.* 1995;19:507-509.
3. Cano N, Labastie-Coeyrehourq J, Lacombe P, et al. Perdialytic parenteral nutrition with lipids and amino acids in malnourished hemodialysis patients. *Am J Clin Nutr.* 1990;52:726-730.
4. Piraino AJ, Firpo JJ, Powers DV. Prolonged hyperalimentation in catabolic chronic dialysis therapy patients. [Review]. *JPEN.* 1981;5:463-477.
5. Pesola GR, Hogg JE, Eissa N, et al. Hypertonic nasogastric tube feedings: do they cause diarrhea? *Crit Care Med.* 1990;18:1073-1079.
6. Cobb DK, High KP, Sawyer RG, at al. A controlled trial of scheduled replacement of central venous and plumonary-artery catheters. *N Engl J Med.* 1992;327:1062-1068.
7. McMahon M, Manji N, Driscoll DF, Bristian BR. Parenteral nutrition in patients with diabetes mellitus: theoretical and practical considerations. *JPEN.* 1989;13:545-553.
8. Makarewicz PA, Freeman JB, Fairfull-Smith R. Prevention of superficial phlebitis during peripheral parenteral nutrition. *Am J Surg.* 1986;151:126-128.
9. Kaminski MV, Williams SD. Review of the rapid normalization of serum albumin with modified total parenteral nutrition solutions. *Crit Care Med.* 1990;18:327-335.
10. Weil MH, Henning RJ, Puri VK. Colloid oncotic pressure: clinical significance. *Crit Care Med.* 1979;7:113-116.
11. Dawidson I, Gelin L, Haglind E. Plasma volume, intravascular protein content, hemodynamic and oxygen transport changes during intestinal shock in dogs. *Crit Care Med.* 1980; 8:73-80.
12. Ford EG, Jennings LM, Andrassy RS. Serum albumin pressure correlates with enteral feeding tolerance in the pediatric surgical patient. *J Ped Surg.* 1987;22:597-599.

13. Zagoren AJ, Weters DW, Beck S, et al. Colloid osmoic pressure: sensitive predictor of enteral feeding tolerance. *JACN.* 1984;3:260.
14. Patterson ML, Dominguez JM, Lymann B, et al. Enteral feeding in the hypoalbuminemic patient. *JPEN.* 1990;14:362-365.
15. Foley EF, Borlase BC, Dzik WH, et al. Albumin-supplementation in the critically ill:A prospective, randomized trial. *Arch Surg.* 1990;125:739-742.
16. Hardin TC, Page CP, Schwesinger WH. Rapid replacement of serum albumin in patients receiving total parenteral nutrition. *Surg Gynecol Obstet.* 1986;163:359-362.
17. Duffy LF, Kerzner B, Gebus V, Dice J. Treatment of central venous occlusions with hydrochloric acid. *J Peds.* 1989;114:1002-1004.
18. Buchman AL, Moukarzel A, Goodson B, et al. Catheter-related infections associated with home parenteral nutrition and predictive factors for the need for catheter removal in their treatment. *JPEN.* 1994;18:297-302.
19. Kim Eh, Cohen RS, Ramachandran P, et al. Adhesion of percutaneously inserted Silastic central venous lines to the vein wall associated with Malassezia furfur infection. *JPEN.* 1993;17:458-460.
20. Solomon SM, Kirby DF. The refeeding syndrome: a review. *JPEN.* 1990;14:90-97.

Suggested Reading

Buchman AL. TPN-associated liver disease. *JPEN.* 2002;26:543-548.

Buchman AL, Morkarzel AA. Metabolic bone disease associated with TPN. *Clin Nutr.* 2000;19:217-231.

Buchman AL. Complications of home total parenteral nutrition. *Dig Dis Sci.* 2001;46:1-28.

Buchman AL, Morkarzel AA, Goodson B, et al. Catheter-related infections associated with home parenteral nutrition and predictive factors for the need for catheter removal in their treatment. *JPEN.* 1994;18:297-302.

Buchman AL, Goodson B, Herzus F, Ament ME. Catheter thrombosis and superior/inferior vena cava syndrome are rare complications of long-term parenteral nutrition. *Clin Nutr.* 1994;13:1356-1360.

Chung C, Buchman AL. TPN-associated and postoperative liver abnormalities. *Liver Clin N Am.* 2002;6:1067-1084.

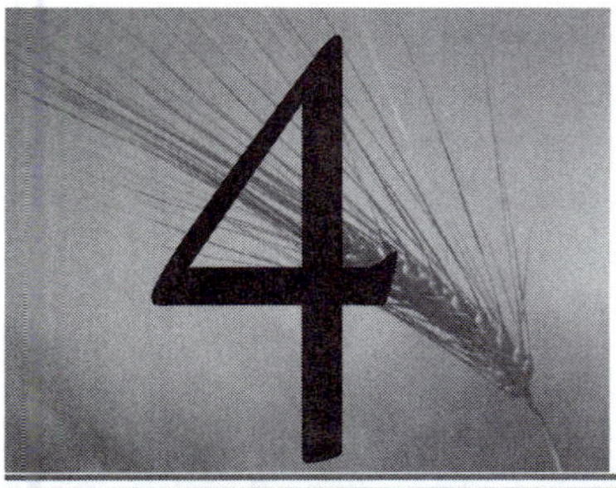

Enteral Nutrition

Transition to Enteral Nutrition

Long-term disuse of the gastrointestinal tract leads to a decrease in villus height after 2 weeks and may lead to intestinal atrophy over long periods. Therefore, when TPN has been used exclusively for more than 2 weeks, the return to oral or enteral (tube feeding) nutrition should be gradual. Parenteral nutrition should be continued until the patient can be 50% to 75% supported with oral or enteral feeding but should be tapered to allow for the hypocaloric stimulation of appetite. The amount of lipid emulsion should be reduced first because it has more effect on appetite suppression and gastric emptying than thalamic controls or dextrose and amino acids.

Tube feeding, when using small bore (8 to 10 FR) nasogastric-feeding tubes, may serve as transitional feeding when parenteral support is being tapered. Enteral nutrition support is preferable to the parenteral route when possible because it is safer, more economical, more nutritionally complete, and maintains gut structure and integrity.

Indications and Contraindications

The old dictum, "if the gut works, use it," still applies. All patients with functioning gastrointestinal tracts who are unable to orally ingest adequate nutrients to meet their nutritional requirements can benefit from supplemental or tube feeding.

Indications include:

1. Protein calorie malnutrition (inadequate oral intake of nutrients for the 5 days prior or normal nutrition status but with inadequate oral intake for the previous 7 to 10 days)
2. Central nervous system (CNS) disorders: comatose state, CVA, Parkinson's disease
3. Neoplasms, especially at least a 2-month prognosis, head and neck carcinoma: nutritional supplementation becomes an ethical concern.

4. Gastrointestinal disease: Crohn's disease, gastroparesis (jejunal feedings), malabsorption, short bowel syndrome (<100 cm jejunum remaining), chronic pancreatitis, possibly severe acute pancreatitis (jejunal feedings), pseudo-obstruction, scleroderma, low output distal enterocutaneous fistuals.
5. Psychiatric disorders: Severe depression, anorexia nervosa.

Contraindications to enteral feeding include:

1. Adynamic ileus
2. Complete intestinal or colonic obstruction
3. Intractable vomiting
4. Proximal high output enterocutaneous fistulas, active gastrointestinal bleeding, and shock. Diarrhea with or without malabsorption may be a contraindication and may possibly be manageable by an adjustment in enteral nutrition flow rate or formula selection.

FEEDING TUBES

Nasoenteric Feeding Tube

Preferably a small bore, 8 to 10 Fr feeding tube should be used. Larger tubes such as the Salem (Kendall, Chicopee, Mass) sump have significant rates of esophageal reflux, ulcer, and stricture formation associated with long-term use, to say nothing of patient discomfort.[1] Risks associated with even small-bore tube placement include pneumomediastinum, bronchopleural fistula, pneumothorax, and hydrothorax. There is no evidence that fine-bore feeding tubes precipitate variceal bleeding in patients with cirrhosis.

Placement should be either in the stomach or the duodenum (or lower). The risk of aspiration is not necessarily decreased with duodenal feeding.[2] However, if duodenal feeding is desired, there is no efficacy in the adjunctive use of metoclopramide, except in the patient with diabetes.[3] However, preliminary studies using erythromycin have suggested the potential benefit of this medication in assuring duodenal placement.

Verify proper tube placement of the tube radiologically before initiating feeding. Physical examination, including auscultatory confirmation, is inaccurate for determining correct tube placement.[4]

Percutaneously Placed or Surgically Placed Gastrostomy Tube

For long-term enteral feeding, gastrostomy tube placement offers no advantages over nasoenteric feeding with respect to patient nutrition, performance, or survival.[5] It eliminates the replacement of the nasoenteric tube every 6 weeks. A percutaneous endoscopic gastrostomy (PEG) tube is less easily dislodged and is more comfortable for the patient. The incidence of nasoesophageal erosion and sinusitis decreases as compared with a nasoenteric feeding tube. There is no decrease in the aspiration risk. Complications do include stomal leakage, tube migration, gastric perforation, bleeding, and wound infection, the latter occurring in <4% of patients.

Jejunostomy tubes require surgical placement, as jejunostomy tubes placed through a PEG invariably flip back into the duodenum or stomach. There are reports of direct percutaneous jejunostomy tube placement, but such a procedure is not accepted at the present time and certainly invites the risk of bowel perforation during the procedure.

Needle-Catheter Jejunostomy

A needle-catheter jejunostomy (NCJ) is easily placed during most abdominal or chest operations and may permit the early introduction of enteral feeding in the hospitalized patient. Catheter dislodgment with intraperitoneal formula leakage occurs in <2% of patients and can be prevented simply by suturing the catheter to the abdominal wall.[6,7] The NCJ is not associated with volvulus or intestinal obstruction.[8] Standard jejunostomy tubes for long-term feeding may also be surgically placed. Endoscopically placed jejunostomy tubes usually migrate back into the stomach or occlude partially because of their small lumens; they are not recommended.

Formula Selection

See Appendix A, Table 46 for a listing of adult enteral formulas and their ingredients.

Considerations

- *Patient diagnosis, nutritional status, and related concerns such as the presence of congestive heart failure, renal or hepatic insufficiency, or hypermetabolic state.*
- *Purpose of the formula.* Oral supplementation where palatability is a concern versus tube feeding where taste is not an issue. Formulas consisting of intact proteins are more palatable (see Enteral Nutrition form, Figure 4-1).
- *Patient's digestive and absorptive ability.* Patients with acute pancreatitis may require feeding with a very low fat containing formula (Vivonex TEN [Novartis, Basel, Switzerland]). Patients with Crohn's disease or malabsorption states may warrant a trial of enteral feeding using a readily available form of protein (free amino acids or short chain peptides) rather than intact protein found in standard formulas. These formulas are substantially more expensive than standard formulas. There is evidence, however, that the use of elemental formulas may not be superior to polymeric formulas in Crohn's disease. Chemically defined formulas are substantially more expensive than standard formulas.
- *Formula osmolality.* The osmolality of a formula may have a direct effect on gastrointestinal side effects and thereby tolerance to enteral therapy. Hyperosmolar formulas have an osmolality of >300 mOsm/kg water. A starter regimen consisting of a diluted formula may be used initially in patients who have had limited oral or enteral nutrient intake in the prior 5 to 7 days. Once the goal rate is achieved, the formula concentration can be increased to full strength. Otherwise, intragastric hyperosmolar formula may precipitate feeding intolerance. Some studies have shown that "starter regimens" are unnec-

essary.[9,10] However, these results may only apply to patients who have had significant recent enteral or oral intake. Jejunal feeding tolerance, on the other hand, is related to the rate of infusion rather than osmolality.

- *Cost*. Specialty formulas cost considerably more than standard isotonic formulas.

Categories of Formulas

Nutritionally Complete Formulas

These formulas are composed of protein, carbohydrate, and fat in high molecular weight form and therefore have lower osmolality. These formulas require normal digestive and lipolytic activity and are also less expensive. Most of these formulas are lactose free and provide 1 kcal/ml. Formulas with higher caloric density (1.5 to 2.0 kcal/ml) are available for use in patients who are fluid restricted. Lower sodium and potassium containing formulas and higher protein containing formulas are also available. Isotonic formulas should *never* be diluted.

Chemically Defined Formulas

These formulas have a low residue and use free amino acids or peptides as a protein source. Oligosaccharides or monosaccharides provide the carbohydrate source and most contain medium as well as long chain triglycerides. These formulas are hyperosmolar, although some are only minimally hyperosmolar and can be infused into the stomach undiluted. Dilution is unnecessary for jejunal feeding. Chemically defined formulas do not require proteolytic capacity, and Vivonex TEN does not require lipolytic activity. Because of the low fat content of Vivonex TEN, exclusive use can lead to essential fatty acid deficiency over an extended period. Theoretically, intestinal absorption of formulas containing di- and tripeptides may be facilitated over those containing crystalline amino acids, although this has not been conclusively demonstrated. In addition, improved absorption does not mean that increased nitrogen will be available for protein synthesis or to improve nitrogen balance.[11] All chemically defined formulas are expensive and should be limited to use in research applications and in patients with malabsorption (fat malabsorption, refractory sprue, extremely short bowel syndrome), pancreatitis, or Crohn's disease.[12,13] Routine use, even in the hypoalbuminemic patient, is unwarranted.[14-16] Routine use of intact protein formulas may actually lead to a lower incidence of diarrhea in postoperative patients who have undergone upper gastrointestinal tract surgery.[17]

Modular Formulas

These formulas are not nutritionally complete because they contain single nutrients such as carbohydrate, fat, or protein. They can be added to standard enteral products but are usually unnecessary and create additional work for food and nutrition services when various complete products are available. Modular formulas include ProMod (Ross, Columbus, Ohio) protein powder (0.2g/ml dry volume or 3 g/tbsp), liquid carbohydrate (0.63 or 2.5 kcal/ml), corn oil (1 g fat containing 0.6 g linoleic acid with 5.4 kcal/ml) and MCT (Mead Johnson, Evansville, Ind) oil (7.7 kcal/ml).

Specialty Formulas

Specialty formulas are available for use in patients with a variety of clinical conditions including renal, respiratory, hepatic insufficiency, diabetes, hypermetabolic states, immunocompromised states, and fat or carbohydrate absorption. There is limited literature describing the use of many of these products. There is even less data supporting the efficacy of many of these formulas. There is limited to no efficacy information available for many of these relatively expensive formulas.[15,18,19] Therefore, careful consideration should be given when contemplating the use of any of these formulas outside of a research setting.

There is also little efficacy for the use of fiber-containing formula even to prevent diarrhea in the critically ill,[20] although this may be related to the use of soy polysaccharide instead of pectin in the formulas. Additional research may yet demonstrate the utility of using fiber-containing formulas in selected patient groups. Soy fiber may improve glucose tolerance.

There is some clinical efficacy in the use of Hepatic-Aid (Hormel, Austin, Minn), a hepatic failure formula (a high-branched chain, low aromatic amino acid containing formula), in chronic hepatic encephalapathy. Patients who would otherwise be unable to ingest a sufficient level of protein without precipitating a worsening of the encephalapathy may benefit from supplementation with this product.[21]

Rate of Administration

Continuous

The volume and rate of formula infusion should be individually determined for each patient based on estimated caloric requirements by equations or indirect calorimetry and estimated protein requirements, confirmed with nitrogen balance studies. Isotonic formulas *never* require dilution. Unless there has been recent prior feeding, continuous drip infusion is preferred over intermittent feedings because initially, a rapid rate of feeding (especially for jejunal feeding) may produce cramping and diarrhea. If there is any question about the patient's digestive and/or absorptive capacity, 24-hour continuous infusion is preferred. To avoid uncontrolled changes in flow rate, an enteral feeding pump is recommended.

Tube feedings into the stomach should be initiated at isotonic strength at a rate of 40 ml/hr. If the patient tolerates this regimen, the rate can then be increased by 25 ml/hr every 8 to 12 hours as tolerated until the prescribed goal is met. Jejunal feeding may require initial rates as low as 10 ml/hr, especially in the immediate postoperative patient. In this situation, gastroparesis may otherwise completely preclude the use of nasogastric feeding. If nausea, vomiting, cramping, or diarrhea occur, the rate of administration should be decreased or, in gastric feedings, the concentration can be decreased. Avoid altering both rate and concentration simultaneously.

Intermittent Feedings

Intermittent feedings can be used if there has been no history of diarrhea or malabsorption, and the gastrointestinal tract is intact.

Bolus Feeding

Bolus infusions can be administered 3 to 5 times daily. They do not require a pump and simulate normal food intake more effectively than continuous feeding, at least in terms of gallbladder motility. Bolus feeding is most useful with a gastrostomy tube and should *never* be used in jejunal feeding. The formula should be administered at a drip rate or via syringe injection not exceeding 240 ml/30 minutes. Use a 100-ml bolus initially and increase the volume by 50 ml daily as tolerated. Orders should be written to specify the number of feedings and the volume to be administered over a specified period. Diarrhea is more common with bolus feeding than with continuous feeding, so consideration must be given to the individual's gastric storage and emptying capacity before considering bolus feeding.[22]

Cyclic, Intermittent Feeding

Like TPN, continuous drip feeding can be compressed or "cycled" into a 10 to 12 overnight feeding. Nighttime feeding may also be used at home for supplemental feeding in patients with active Crohn's disease or other malabsorption conditions. The patient or significant other is trained to intubate their stomach with a nasoenteric tube nightly. In most cases, this is not recommended because of the possibility of improper tube placement. Night time feeding may also be used with gastrostomy but not with jejunostomy tube feeding.

Fluid Requirements

No formula provides sufficient free water to meet a patient's daily fluid requirement. The recommended daily water requirement in the absence of hepatic, renal, or cardiac disease is 1/ml/kcal. Most 1 kcal/ml formulas contain approximately 75% water. Therefore, patients without fluid restriction should receive enough additional free water to equal at least 25% of the total formula volume (ie, for 2000 ml of formula per 24 hours, an additional 500 ml of water is required). The additional free water can be administered in 2 or 3 divided doses. The water used to flush the tube from feedings or medications should be included in this total. Tap water is fine; distilled water is unnecessary.

Monitoring

Proper monitoring of patients receiving enteral nutrition is necessary to detect and prevent complications.

1. Confirm placement of feeding tube by radiograph before initiating feeding. Studies have revealed the inaccuracy of auscultation or aspiration.[23] If the feeding tube becomes dislodged, proper placement should be re-verified by radiograph.
2. Keep the patient's head and shoulders (not solely only the head of the bed) elevated at 30 to 45 degrees at all times during feeding and for 1 hour after feeding is completed to prevent aspiration of the formula.
3. Use a 30 to 35 ml syringe to check gastric residuals every 4 hours. The residual should be 150 ml. If not, the feeding should be held and the condition investigated. If residual is 150 ml, return contents to stomach. Gastric residuals may be difficult to obtain if small bore nasogastric tubes are used because the negative suction induced by the syringe will collapse the tube. Gastric residuals may be increased due to delayed gastric emptying caused by recent adminis-

tration of hypertonic medications in liquid form. After checking the gastric residual, the tube should be flushed with 30 ml of water to avoid clogging. Checking residuals is not useful for jejunal feeding because they do not accurately reflect jejunal emptying. Avoid the use of 30-ml syringes because injection force when returning the residual may be sufficient to rupture the tube and cause tissue damage.

4. Maintain accurate intake and output records and record the amount of prescribed feeding actually received.
5. Record patient's weight at least 3 times weekly.
6. Observe the patient for abdominal distention, pain, diarrhea, or dyspnea and treat accordingly.

Monitor the patient's response to therapy at least:

Every 8 hours	Vital signs
Twice weekly	Electrolytes including Mg, Ca, P, blood glucose, BUN, creatinine
Biweekly	Total protein, albumin, prealbumin, CBC with differential, AST, ALT

Monitoring frequency may be decreased in stable, long-term enterally fed patients (Figure 4-1).

Complications of Enteral Feeding

Mechanical

Obstruction of the Tube Lumen

Flush the tube with 30 ml of water every 4 to 6 hours, after discontinuing enteral feeding and following the administration of medications through the tube to prevent any clogging of the feeding tube. Some medications are not compatible with enteral feeding and will lead to precipitation in the tube. Sucralfate should never be administered through a nasogastric feeding tube.

Protocol for Treating a Clogged Feeding Tube

Attempt to flush the tube with warm water using only mild pressure to avoid rupturing the tube. Use only finger pressure on the plunger.

Unclogging Enteric Feeding Tubes

1. Use:
   A. Sugar-free, decaffeinated soda (does not require physician order).
   B. Meat tenderizer (papain). Mix 1 teaspoon non-potato flake papain meat tenderizer with the smallest amount of tap water required for dissolving.
   C. Pancrease (Ortho-McNeil, Raritan, NJ) or Viokase (Paddock Laboratories, Minneapolis, Minn) (pancreatic enzyme). Mix 1 crushed pancreas enzyme tablet (Amylase 30,000 units, Protease 13,000 units, and Lipase 8,000 units per tablet) with 1 crushed tablet (324 mg) sodium bicarbonate and 5 ml tap

Northwestern University Medical Center
676 N. St. Clair Street Chicago, Ill 60611

Check Box: ☐ **Initiation Order** ☐ **Rate change only ______ mL/hr** ☐ **New Order**

ESTIMATED NEEDS	**Height ____ Current Weight ___ kg Ideal Body Weight __ kg** Estimated caloric requirement __________ kcal/day Estimated protein requirement __________ kcal/day ☐ **Check box** to order **Indirect Calorimetry** to determine resting energy expenditure
ROUTE OF ADMINISTRATION	**Check one box:** ☐ Nasoenteric ☐ Gastrostomy ☐ Jejunostomy

FORMULA					
		ISOTONIC (Osmolite)	**ISOTONIC HN (Osmolite HN)**	**ISOTONIC HIGH FIBER (Jevity)**	**CONCENTRATED (Two Cal HN)**
	non-protein kcal/ml **kcal/ml** **total protein g/L**	0.91 1.06 36	0.89 1.06 44.4	0.93 1.06 44.5	1.69 2.01 83.4
		HIGH FAT/LOW CARB (Pulmocare)	**HYDROLYZED PROTEIN (ELEMENTAL) (Vital HN)**	**FREE AMINO ACID (ELEMENTAL) (Vivonex)**	**HIGH FIBER HIGH FAT/LOW CARB (Glucerna)**
	non-protein kcal/ml **kcal/ml** **total protein g/L**	1.26 1.5 62.6	0.64 1.0 41.7	0.85 1.0 38.2	0.89 1.0 41.8
		Renal (Suplena)	**Renal (dialysis) (Nepro)**	**Hepatic Failure (Nutrihep)**	
	non-protein kcal/ml **kcal/ml** **total protein g/L**	1.88 2.0 29.9	1.72 2.0 69.6	1.35 1.5 40	

☐ Other Nutrient Components — Check box and complete if necessary:

DIRECTIONS, INFUSING RATE, AND MONITORING

Administration method: (circle A or B). Fill in blanks.

A. **Continuous Administration**
1) Confirm tube position by x-ray before tube is used (upper abdominal x-ray for tube placement)
2) Initiate half/full **(circle one)** strength at ________ mL/hr.
3) Check gastric residuals q.4h. If residual >150 ml, hold feeding and notify M.D.
4) Elevate patient's head & shoulders 30-45E at all times during feeding & for 60 minutes after feeding is stopped.
5) Advance feeding by _____ ml every ____ hrs to a goal rate of _____ mL/hr. Once goal rate is achieved, advance to full strength after _____ hrs (does not apply to isotonic or jejunal feeding).
6) Do not stop feeding for postural drainage if patient has an endotracheal or tracheostomy tube in place with an inflated cuff.
7) Rinse feeding tube with 30 ml tap water q.4h.

B. **Cyclic or Bolus Administration** (bolus administration not recommended for J-tube feeding)
1) Confirm tube position by x-ray before tube is used (nasoenteric feeding only).
2) Gravity drop at half/full (circle one) strength feeding, ____ ml over 30 minutes q.____ hrs.
3) Check gastric residual prior to each feeding. If residual >150 ml, hold feeding and notify M.D. Do not check residuals for duodenal or jejunostomy feeding. Signs of intolerance may include nausea, vomiting, abdominal pain or distention, diarrhea.
4) Keep patient's head and shoulders elevated 30-45E at all times during feeding and for 60 minutes after feeding is stopped.
5) Rinse feeding tube with 30 ml tap water after each feeding.

The following will be performed unless otherwise ordered:
Nutrition panel I (electrolytes, glucose, BUN, creat, Ca, Mg, P) qOD x3 then q.Mon.
Nutrition panel II (alb, pre-alb, total protein, LFTs) q.Mon
Weigh patient M.W.F., Daily I and O

Date/Time Written: __________ Time/Date Noted: __________ Physician Signature: __________ Physician (Dictation) I.D. #:	ADDRESSOGRAPH:

Figure 4-1. Adult enteral nutrition orders.

water to prepare a pancreatic solution. Allow it to sit for 5 minutes to activate enzyme.

2. Check tube position, preferably by chest or abdominal x-ray.
3. Severe lung damage can occur if the declogging solution is administered into the bronchial tree.
4. Elevate the head and shoulders of the patient's bed to an upright, or at least 45-degree angle.
5. Clear an obstructed feeding tube as soon as possible.
6. Before using any solution to declog the tubing, aspirate very slowly as much liquid from the tube as possible using a 30 to 50 ml catheter tip or Luer-lock syringe.
7. Instill 5 ml or more of one of the declogging solutions using a 30 to 50 ml syringe. Use of water or soda should be attempted first to unclog tubes.
8. Clamp the tube and wait 15 minutes.
9. Then try to aspirate or flush the tube with water.
10. The procedure may need to be repeated (repeat steps 2 and 3).
11. Meat tenderizer and pancreatic enzyme solutions may be more effective than water or soda.
    A. Papain-containing meat tenderizer should be obtained from the pharmacy or food service.

Esophageal Complications

- Esophagitis, erosions, ulceration, stricture or mucosal bridge function.
- More common with the use of larger tubes such as Ryle's-type or Salem sump. Avoid these types of tubes for enteral feeding.

Nasopharyngeal Complications

- Discomfort usually minor and self-limited with small-bone tubes, but short-term use of an analgesic or anesthetic lozenges may be helpful.
- Nasal erosions and sloughing of nasal cartilage may result from excessive pressure on the nasal alae and nasal cartilage. Nasoenteric tubes should be routinely changed to the opposite nares after no more than 4 to 6 weeks.
- If long-term enteral feeding (>4 to 6 weeks) is required, a PEG or percutaneous endoscopic jejunostomy (PEJ) should be placed.
- Otitis media and/or sinusitis may occur because of occlusion of sinus tracts or the eustachian tube related to pressure from the nasoenteric feeding tube. All patients who have a nasoenteric tube end are connected to a ventilator should be routinely examined with an octoscope.

Rupture of Esophageal Varices

- Does *not* occur with the use of small bore feeding tubes.

Tracheoesophageal Fistula

- Usually occurs with a large bone tube and a concurrent nasotracheal or tracheostomy tube.
- Caused by pressure necrosis and erosion through the posterior tracheal wall into the anterior wall of the esophagus.

Tube Misplacement

- Tube position should be verified by *radiograph* before initiating feeding, or should the tube become dislodged. Auscultation may not indicate if the tube has been placed in the pleural space, lung, or pharynx in an unconscious patient.[23]
- The guidewire should *never* be replaced in a nasoenteric feeding tube still inside the patient. The wire may exit the tube in an inappropriate location and result in esophageal or sinus perforation.
- In the situation where a nasoenteric feeding tube is dislodged or removed by a disoriented patient, a nasal bridle can be used to secure the tube.[24]

Complications of PEG/PEJ

1. Wound infections
   - A. Cellutitis at tube skin exit site
   - B. Abdominal abscess
   - C. May be prevented by the use of prophylactic antibiotics, although this may be of little help.[25]
   - D. Necrotizing fasciitis may rarely occur if an abdominal wall infection is not recognized promptly.
2. Leakage around tube
   - A. A small amount of secretion at the skin exit site is normal; leakage may require tube replacement with a larger sized tube.
3. Bleeding from the puncture site
4. Premature removal by patient
   - A. May cause separation of the stomach and anterior abdominal wall if removed within 10 to 14 days of placement. Keep patient nothing by mouth (NPO) and perform a water-soluble contrast study to evaluate for extravasation. A gastric leak usually requires surgical repair. After 10 to 14 days the tube can usually be replaced percutaneously. However, the gastrocutaneous fistula may often close within 24 hours. Proper position within the gastric lumen should be documented before restarting feeding.
5. Gastrocolic fistula (PEG only)
   - A. Rare, usually recognized a month or more after insertion
   - B. Usually results with PEG removal
6. Gastric outlet obstruction (PEG only)
   - A. Caused by tube migration

   B. Occurs more frequently with foley catheter replacement tubes because there is no external skin bolster to prevent distal tube migration.
7. Gastroesophageal reflux (PEG only)
   A. May be related to reduced lower esophageal sphincter pressure.
8. Excessive granulation tissue (at the skin site exit)
   A. May be painful.
   B. Treated by application of silver nitrate-impregnated cue tips.
9. Visceral perforation
   A. Avoid placement if transilluminator of endoscope light is not clear.

PEG/PEJ Maintenance

It is important to keep the PEG site clean and dry; occlusive dressings are unnecessary and may increase bacterial contamination because of the resultant moist environment.

Skin Irritation

- Usually related to leakage of gastric contents.
- May be prevented by avoiding the use of occlusive dressings and keeping the PEG exit site clean and dry.

Gastrostomy		Jejunostomy	
Advantages	*Disadvantages*	*Advantages*	*Disadvantages*
Can be placed w/o surgery.	Does not decrease risk of aspiration related to delayed gastric emptying.	Reduces risk of aspiration in cases of delayed gastric emptying unsuccessful. No risk of GE reflux may allow more immediate post-operative feeding.	Requires surgery (endoscopically placed) PEG usually in the long-term. Cannot use bolus feedings.

Gastrointestinal Complications

Sudden nausea, vomiting, or diarrhea that develops after initiation of tube feeding may be due to:

1. Improper formula temperature
2. Irregular or too rapid administration of formula
3. Bacterial contamination of the formula
   A. To avoid bacterial contamination of formula it is necessary to hang formula bags no longer than 4 hours and to change the feeding bag and tubing every 24 hours. Closed systems can be hung for 24 hours.
4. Bacterial overgrowth in the bowel
5. Hyperosmolar reactions to a formula with high osmolality when hyperosmolar formulas are infused into the stomach
   A. Even diets >700mOsm can be well tolerated when infused into the stomach if infused slowly with a pump.

6. Concurrent medication

Most diarrhea associated with enteral feeding is usually caused by concurrent antibiotics or sorbitol as part of oral solutions.[26] Nearly all formulas are lactose free. Pesola et al[27] showed that hypertonic feeding (690 mOsm) infused into the stomach in postoperative head and neck cancer patients with a mean serum albumin concentration of 2.8g/dl did not necessarily result in diarrhea.

If diarrhea develops, and is presumed secondary to the enteral feeding, the rate of feeding should first be decreased until the diarrhea resolves. If readvancement of the rate is not possible, loperamide should be administered. If this is unsuccessful, paregoric (5 to 20 ml) can be added to each 8-hour feeding formula volume or administered as a bolus every 4 hours through the feeding tube.

Gallstones may also develop because of impaired CCK release and gallbladder dysmotility. This problem can be avoided by the use of cyclic or bolus feeding.

Pulmonary Aspiration

Transpyloric feeding tube placement does not necessarily reduce the risk of aspiration of formula into the lungs.[2]

The cause for aspiration pneumonia in patients who are enterally fed that have suffered CNS insults is largely aspiration of posterior pharyngeal secretions. This cannot be prevented by head elevation and if it occurs is usually unrelated to enteral feeding.

Metabolic Complications

The most common electrolyte abnormalities encountered in patients receiving tube feeding are hypernatremia, hyponatremia, hypercalcemia, and azotemia. These complications can often be prevented by proper monitoring of fluid intake, hydration status, and adjustment of the electrolyte content of the formula. Hyperosmotic metabolic alkalosis will result if insufficient free water is provided. Complications of overfeeding and the refeeding syndrome may also occur with enteral feeding.

Home Enteral Feeding

The patient or significant other must be trained in the use of enteral feeding, nasoenteric, gastrostomy or jejunostomy feeding tubes, site care (PEG or jejunostomy), and use of an enteral feeding pump (if necessary). Sufficient time for patient training should be allowed before discharge.

References

1. Cabre E, Gonzalez-Huix F, Abad-Lacruz A, et al. Effect of total enteral nutrition on the short-term outcome of severely malnourished cirrhotics. *Gastroenterology.* 1990;18:327-335.
2. Strong RM, Condon SC, Solinger MR, et al. Equal aspiration rates from postpylorus and intragastric-placed small-bore nasoenteric feeding tubes: a randomized, prospective study. *JPEN.* 1992;16:59-63.
3. Kittinger JW, Sandler RS, Heizer WD. Efficiency of metoclopramide as an adjunct to duodenal placement of small-bore feeding tubes: a randomized, placebo-controlled, double-blind study. *JPEN.* 1987;11:33-7.
4. Woodhall BH, Winfield DF, Bisset GS. Inadvertent tracheobronchial placement of feeding tubes. *Radiology.* 1987;165:727-729.
5. Fay DE, Poplausky M, Gruber, M, Lance P. Long-term enteral feeding: a retrospective comparison of delivery via percutaneous endoscopic gastrostomy and nasoenteric tubes. *Am J Gastroenterol.* 1991;86:1604-1609.
6. Page CP. Needle catheter jejunostomy. *Contemp Surg.* 1981;19:47.
7. Schattenkerk ME, Obertop H, Bruining A, et al. Early postoperative enteral feeding by a needle catheter jejunostomy after 100 esophageal resections and reconstructions for cancer. *Clin Nutr.* 1984;47.
8. Ryan JA Jr, Page CP. Intrajejunal feeding: development and current status. *JPEN.* 1984;8:187.
9. Keohane PP, Attrill H, Love M, et al. Relation between osmolality of diet and gastrointestinal side effects of enteral nutrition. *Br Med J.* 1984;288:678-80.
10. Rees RG, Keohane PP. Elemental diet administered nasogastrically without starter regimens to patients with inflammatory bowel disease. *JPEN.* 1986;10:258-62.
11. Steinhardt HS, Wolf A, Jakobr B, et al. Protein assimilation in pancreatectomized patients: efficiency of absorption from whole versus hydrolyzed protein. *Gastroenterology.* 1986;90:1648.
12. Adibi SA, Fogel MR, Agrawal RM. Comparison of free amino acid and dipeptide absorption in the jejunum of sprue patients. *Gastroenterology.* 1974; 67: 586-591.
13. Vazquez JA, Morse EL, Adibi SA. Effect of starvation on amino acid and peptide transport and peptide by hydrolysis in humans. *Am J Physiol.* 1985;294:G563-G566.
14. Koretz RL, Meyer JH. Elemental diets-facts and fantasies. *Gastroenterology.* 1980;78:393-410.
15. Mowatt-Larssen CA, Brown RO, Wojtsysiak SL, et al. Comparison of tolerance and nutritional outcome between a peptide and a standard enteral formula in critically ill, hypoalbuminemic patients. *JPEN.* 1992;16:20-24.
16. Silk DB. Diet formulation and choice of enteral diet. *Gut.* 1986;27:40-6.
17. Kemen M, Homann HH, Mumme A, et al. Is intact protein similar for postoperative enteral nutrition than hydrolyzed protein? *Clin Nutr.* 1991;10:37S.
18. Ford EG, Hull SF, Jennings LM, Andrassy RJ. Clinical comparison of tolerance to elemental or polymeric enteral feedings in the postoperative patient. *JACN.* 1992;11:11-16.
19. Rees RG, Harp WR, Grimble GK, Frost PG, Silk DB. Do patients with moderately impaired gastrointestinal function requiring enteral nutrition need a predigested nitrogen source? *Gut.* 1992;33:877-81.
20. Dobb GJ, Towler SC. Diarrhea during enteral feeding in the critically ill: a comparison of feeds with and without fiber. *Intens Care Med.* 1990;16:252-5.

21. Comparison of dietary protein with an oral, branched chain-enriched amino acid supplement on chronic portal-systemic encephalography. *Hepatology.* 1984;4:279-87.
22. Heitkemper ME, Martin DL, Hansen BC, et al. Rate and volume of intermittent enteral feeding. *JPEN.* 1981;5:125-9.
23. Metheny N. Measures to test placement of nasogastric and nosintestinal feeding tubes: a review. *Nurs Res.* 1988;37:324-9.
24. Meer JA. A new nasal bridle for securing nasenteral feeding tubes. *JPEN.* 1989;13:331-334.
25. Jonas SK, Neimark S, Panwalker AP. Effect of antibiotic prophylaxis in percutaneous endoscopic gastrostomy. *Am J Gastroenterol.* 1985;80:438.
26. Edes TE, Walk BE, Austin JL. Diarrhea in tube-fed patients: feeding formula not necessarily the cause. *Am J Med.* 1990;88:91-3.
27. Pesola GR, Hogg JE, Eisssa N, et al. Hypertonic nasogastric tube feedings: do they cause diarrhea? *Crit Care Med.* 1990;18:1378-82.

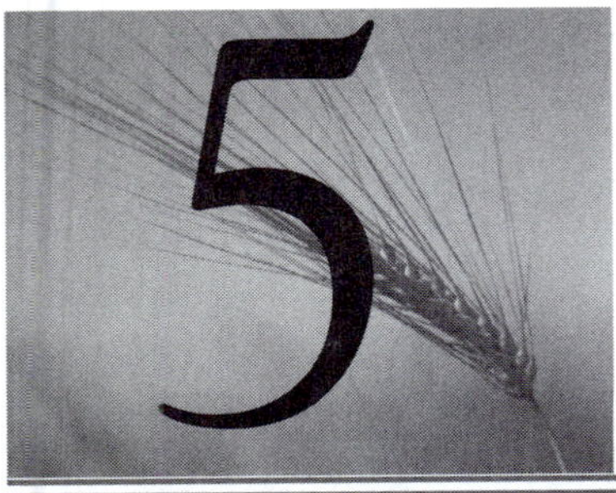

5 Pediatric Nutritional Support

Timothy A. Sentongo, MD

Growth and nutritional status in children are important indicators of health and well-being. Therefore, nutrition assessment is an integral part of the evaluation of all children, particularly those with chronic illness and/or impaired growth. Malnutrition encompasses both being overweight and failure to thrive. Growth and nutritional disturbances occur in feeding disorders, acute and chronic illness, and during prolonged hospitalization, particularly when oral intake is suspended or limited. Nutritional support requires assessment of nutritional status, severity of malnutrition and monitoring of the response to intervention. This is accomplished by careful and repeated measurements of growth, nutritional status, energy requirements, and response to nutritional intervention.

History and Physical Examination

History and physical examination are of primary importance and should include:

- A 3-day diet diary that is analyzed by a dietician.
- Unusual dietary habits such as fad vegetarian, participation in sports with weight-based classes, intentional weight loss, or lipid lowering diets.
- Any medications (Appendix A, Table 43).
- History should screen for potential etiology for impaired growth—ie, organic versus non-organic failure to thrive (Appendix C, Table 1).
- Careful physical examination may suggest specific nutrient deficiencies. Therefore examination of hair, skin, teeth, mucous membranes, nails, distribution of body fat and muscle mass is very important (Appendix A, Table 1).
- Presence of digital clubbing (convex nail plates) may suggest chronic disease—eg, cystic fibrosis, liver disease, and chronic inflammatory bowel disease.

Growth and Nutritional Assessment

- Proper instruments, carefully obtained measurements, and suitable reference data are essential for meaningful assessment of growth and nutritional status.
- Age- and situation-appropriate time intervals should be selected between growth measurements (Table 5-1).
- Pubertal status should also be assessed because of its effect on interpretation of growth status and potential. See Appendix B, Figures 18 and 19.

Weight

- The updated 2000 Centers for Disease Control and Prevention (CDC) weight-for-age growth charts for healthy children aged birth to 20 years should be used. See Appendix B, Figures 1 through 4.
- Online provisions are also available to compute individualized growth percentiles and standard deviation scores (z-scores). See www.cdc.gov/growthcharts.
- Tanner-Whitehouse weight velocity charts may be used to monitor rate of weight gain in girls aged 1 to 16 years and boys aged 1 to 17 years. See Appendix B, Figures 7 and 8.
- Premature infant growth reference charts for weight, length, and head circumference are also available. See Appendix B, Figure 9.
- Online individualized premature infant growth reference charts may be accessed at: www.neonatal.rti.org. Use requires Microsoft Internet Explorer.
- Down syndrome weight-for-age growth reference charts. See Appendix B, Figures 10 through 13.

Stature (Length and Height)

Measuring linear growth is important for assessing growth status, interpretation of weight, and screening for disease and malnutrition (being overweight and failure to thrive). Appropriate equipment and technique are critical for obtaining accurate and reliable measurements. For purposes of accuracy, it is recommended that all measurements should be repeated and an average obtained.[1]

- Length (supine) is measured to the nearest 0.1 cm in children younger than 2 to 3 years or older children who cannot stand. Length should be assessed using a length board (stadiometer) or firm surface. It requires 2 measurers: one to position the head and the other to stretch and straighten the legs so that the knees are flat and feet at a 90-degree angle with the footboard.
- Standing height is measured to the nearest 0.1 cm after age 2 years in children able to evenly support their weight on both feet. It is obtained with bare feet, and heels, buttocks, shoulders, and back of head should be against the measuring device and with eyes looking straight ahead.
- The updated 2000 CDC length/height-for-age growth charts for healthy children aged birth to 20 years should be used. See Appendix B, Figures 1 through 4.

TABLE 5-1

Recommended Time Intervals for Growth Measurements

Measurement	Initial Period	Long-Term Follow-Up
Weight	Daily (preterm infants to age ≤1-y) Twice a week (age > 1-y)	2 to 4 weeks 1 to 3 months
Length	7 days (preterm infants)	4 weeks
Height	4 weeks	1 to 6 months
Head Circumference	7 days (preterm infants)	4 weeks (age <3 y)
Mid-Arm Circumference	4 weeks	1 to 6 months
Triceps skinfold	4 weeks	1 to 6 months

- Online provisions are also available to compute individualized length/height percentiles and standard deviation scores (z-scores) based on the 2000 CDC growth charts. See www.cdc.gov/growthcharts.
- Tanner-Whitehouse height velocity charts may be used to monitor rate of height gain in girls aged 1 to 16 years and boys aged 1 to 19 years. See Appendix B, Figures 5 and 6.
    - Height below the 5th percentile indicates short stature. Height velocity below the 5th percentile suggests severely stunted growth that warrants assessment of pubertal status and screening of for familial stature; constitutional growth delay; malnutrition; and organic disorders including chronic inflammatory diseases, endocrine, skeletal, and genetic disorders.
- Premature infant growth reference charts for weight, length, and head circumference are also available. See Appendix B, Figure 9.
- Online individualized premature infant growth reference charts may be accessed at: www.neonatal.rti.org. Use requires Microsoft Internet Explorer.
- Down syndrome length- and height-for-age growth reference charts are available. See Appendix B, Figures 10 through 13.
- For children who are bedridden or with spinal kyphoscoliosis, extremity contractures, and other forms of musculoskeletal deformities preventing accurate measurement of stature may be assessed using upper arm and lower limb lengths.[1] Measurement requires training in anthropometry and special instruments (anthropometer). See upper arm and lower limb growth reference charts for girls aged 3 to 16 years and boys aged 3 to 18 years. Appendix B, Figures 20 through 23.

Head Circumference

- Is useful until age 3 years, after which the velocity of head growth slows.
- Must be measured with a non-stretchable measuring tape. Anteriorly the tape is placed just superior to the eyebrows and posteriorly it is placed so that the maximum circumference is measured.
- Reference values from birth to age 3 years (see Appendix B, Figures 14 and 15).
- Premature infant reference values (see Appendix B, Figure 9).

Interpretation of Weight-for-Length Growth Indices

Weight-for-length percentiles provide a means of assessing a child's weight while taking into account their length.[1,2] See 2000 CDC weight-for-length growth reference charts for children aged birth to 36 months. Appendix B, Figures 14 and 15.

- High (>90th percentile) weight-for-length percentile indicates increased body weight in relation to length suggestive of overweight status.
- High weight-for-length percentile combined with low length-for-age percentile suggests a non-nutritional etiology for short stature. Children with this pattern of growth should be considered for evaluation for familial short stature, and genetic, endocrine, and skeletal disorders.
- Decreased weight-for-length (<5th percentile) is suggestive of nutritional wasting, which may be primary (non-organic) or secondary to gastrointestinal or other systemic disease (see Appendix C, Table 1). Children with negative energy balance from inadequate caloric intake, acute malnutrition, chronic illness or malabsorption have a decreased weight-for-length percentile (ie, are abnormally thin). In chronically malnourished children, weight loss precedes impaired linear growth, which in turn precedes decreased head growth (in children aged <3 years).
- Children with disproportionately small heads may have primary neurological problems affecting brain growth, because head growth is the last to be affected by primary malnutrition and is not characteristic of primary skeletal disorders.

Percent Ideal Body Weight

- Calculated by dividing the actual weight by the ideal weight for the child's height multiplied by 100. The ideal body weight is defined as the median weight for the child's length/height.

Under nutrition	90%
Severe marasmus	75% (<65% requires hospitalization)
Overweight	>110%
Obese	>120%

Body Mass Index

Body mass index (BMI) kg/m^2 is a weight-stature index computed by dividing body weight in kg by height squared in meters ($weight/height^2$). BMI is very useful for screening, monitoring and early intervention in children and adolescents who are overweight (95th percentile) or at risk for being overweight (85th percentile and <95th percentile). Similarly BMI may be used to assess being underweight or risk for being underweight. 2000 CDC BMI-for-age growth reference charts for children and adolescents aged 2 to 20 years are available. BMI does not distinguish between overweight status from excess body fat versus increased muscularity, edema, or ascites. Therefore measuring body fat stores using triceps skinfold (TSF) will improve accuracy. Computing BMI z-score is also available online at: www.cdc.gov/growthcharts. See BMI growth charts in Appendix B, Figures 16 and 17.

Anthropometry

Mid-upper-arm circumference (MAC) and TSF are very practical and useful for assessing nutritional status and monitoring short- and long-term response to nutritional support and intervention. Good reference data is available for several anthropometry measurements. Training is required for reliable and reproducible measurements. Proper techniques are described in *Anthropometric Standardization Reference Manual*, edited by Lohman et al (1988 Champaign, Ill: Human Kinetics).

Mid-Upper-Arm Circumference

- Is a composite measure of muscle, fat, and bone.
- It should be obtained using a non-stretchable measuring tape. Measurements are taken from either arm at the mid-point between the acromion or shoulder and olecranon or elbow.
- Reference values and percentiles are available for healthy children, adolescents, and adults. See Appendix A, Table 3.

Mid-Arm Circumference to Head Circumference Ratio

- Reflects weight for length.
- Useful when apparatus for measuring weight or length is not available.
- Useful only up to 3 years of age when head growth slows.
- Reference values shown in Figure 5-1.

Triceps Skinfold Thickness

- Measures body fat.
- Very good indicator of the body's energy reserves.

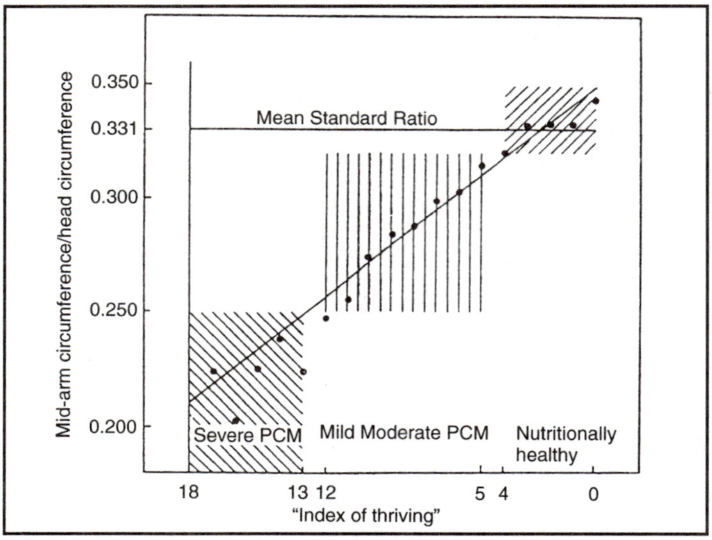

Figure 5-1. Mid-arm circumference to head circumference ratio compared with an "index of thriving" based on weight, height, head circumference, and mid-arm circumference in protein-calorie malnutrition (PCM). (Reprinted with permission from Kanawate A, McLaren DS. Assessment of marginal malnutrition. *Nature*. 1970;228:573-574. Copyright 1970 Macmillan Magazines Limited.

- Measurement requires skinfold caliper and training in anthropometry.
- Changes rapidly with change in nutritional status.
- Correlates very well with the body's fat stores.
- Good reference data available for ages 1 to adulthood. See Appendix A, Table 6.

Upper Arm Muscle Area, mm²

- Index for estimating muscle stores.
- MAC is combined with TSF to calculate upper arm muscle area:

Upper-arm muscle area, mm² = $[MAC - (TSF \times \pi)]^2/(4 \times \pi)$
$\pi = 3.14$; Multiply MAC, cm by 10 to convert to mm

- Reference values are available for upper arm muscle area in children aged 1 to adulthood. See Appendix C, Table 2.
  Example: 3-year-old male child
  Arm circumference = 16.4 cm; Triceps skinfold = 10.3 mm
  Multiple MAC, cm by 10 to convert to mm
  Upper arm muscle area
  $[164 - (10.3 \times 3.14)]^2/4 \times 3.14 = 1339$ mm² (10th to 25th percentile)

Body Composition

- *Weight* is a composite measure of the body's fat-free mass (lean tissue and bone) and fat mass (adipose tissue). *Lean body mass* is indicative of water and protein content of the body. *Fat tissue* represents the body's energy stores. *Bone mass* represents the calcium and mineral stores. *Lean tissue* (muscle) is depleted during

TABLE 5-2

Comparison of the Time, Expense, Practicality, and Accuracy of Body Composition Methods in Children

Method	Time	Expense	Practicality in Infants	Practicality in Older Children	Accuracy	Available Reference Data
Anthropometry	+	++	+/-	+++	+/-	++
TOBEC	++	--	+/-	++	+	-
BIA	++	+	-	+	-	-
Isotope Dilution $2H_2O$	+	-	+++	+++	+++	-
DXA	+	+/-	+	++	+++	+
K-40	---	---	---	--	?	-
Neutron Activation	--	---	--	--	+++	-

+ represents relative advantage - represents relative disadvantage

states of chronic malnutrition, cachexia, and inactivity. During health fat tissue is laid down when there is *positive energy balance* (energy intake in excess of expenditure for basal metabolism, growth, physical activity and losses). Bone mineralization may be impaired during malnutrition, delayed skeletal maturity, chronic illness, and medications. Weight and stature may be stable; however, these body compartments change differently during *growth* (infancy, childhood, and puberty); chronic illness; malnutrition; and nutritional rehabilitation. Therefore, assessing body composition provides more detailed information about nutritional status than weight or stature alone.[1]

- Many methods to measure body composition exist, but most have limited clinical application. The most available and frequently used method is anthropometry (combined weight, stature, and skinfolds). The other methods include total body electrical conductivity (TOBEC), bioelectrical impedance analysis (BIA), hydrodensitometry (underwater weighing), total body water (isotope dilution), dual body x-ray absorptiometry (DXA), computerized axial tomography (CAT Scan), total body potassium (K-40), and neutron activation (Table 5-2).

Laboratory Assessment

- The initial laboratory evaluation of nutritional status includes assessment of hematological and visceral protein status. Commonly measured visceral proteins and their half-lives are listed in Table 5-3.
- Serum values of visceral proteins may not reflect the degree of nutritional deficiency because during chronic malnutrition and starvation there is a tendency to preserve the circulating pool of visceral proteins at the expense of somatic protein.

TABLE 5-3

Half Lives of Serum Proteins

Albumin	20 days
Transferrin	8 days
Prealbumin (Transthyretin)	2 days
Retinol binding protein	10 hours

- Appendix A, Table 30 shows normal values for various biochemical measurements commonly used to evaluate nutritional status in children.
- Immune function is reflected in total lymphocyte count and presence of anergy by skin testing.

NUTRITIONAL REQUIREMENTS

Fluid

MAINTENANCE FLUID REQUIREMENTS FOR CHILDREN

Holiday-Sega Method:[3,4]

- Fluid and electrolyte requirements are based on metabolic rate. It is recommended that for every 100 kcal expended, 100 ml of water should be administered. Therefore the Holliday-Sega method determines fluid requirements based on estimated caloric expenditure calculated from body weight. Not suitable for preterm infants, neonates age <14 days, or conditions associated with abnormal fluid losses or retention (Table 5-4).
- Caloric expenditure and therefore fluid requirement is increased by fever (12%/°Celsius rise in body temperature) and by hypermetabolic states such as salicylism and hyperthyroidism (25% to 75%). Likewise, it is decreased by hypothermia (12%/°Celsius fall in body temperature) and by hypometabolic states such as hypothyroidism (10% to 25%).

Additional fluid requirements in the dehydrated child can be estimated from Table 5-5 or from actual weight loss.

- Oral rehydration solutions (ORS) contain a mixture of sodium and glucose. Their mechanism of effect involves absorption of sodium and glucose via the ATP-independent Na+-coupled glucose cotransporter into the apical villous cells. This causes an osmotic gradient resulting in passive diffusion of water from the intestinal lumen into the enterocyte.
- Oral solutions used for *rehydration* should contain 75 to 90 mEq/L of sodium. In contrast solutions used for *prevention* of dehydration or maintenance of hydration status should contain 40 to 60 mEq/L of sodium.[5] Composition of oral electrolyte solutions are shown in the Table 5-6.

TABLE 5-4

Holliday-Sega Method

Body Weight, kg	Maintenance Fluid Requirements/Day
Up to 10	100 cc/kg
11 to 20	1,000 cc + 50 cc/kg for each kg above 10 kg
> 20	1,500 cc + 20 cc/kg for each kg above 20 kg

TABLE 5-5

Clinical Signs of Dehydration

2 to 3%	thirst, mild oliguria
5 to 6%	thirst, oliguria, slightly sunken fontanel in infants, thick, tenacious saliva, slight decrease in skin turgor, slightly sunken eyes
7 to 8%	marked thirst and oliguria, sunken fontanel, dry mouth, obvious loss of skin turgor (hypertonic dehydration causes thick, doughy skin), sunken eyes with decreased intraocular tension, restlessness or apathy
>10%	as above; thirst may be lost; peripheral vasoconstriction, hypotension, cyanosis, occasional fever, increased respiratory rate (hypertonic dehydration may cause irritability and seizures)

MILD DEHYDRATION: <5%

- Rehydration: ORS 40 ml/kg over 4 hours
- Maintenance: Resume regular formula or lactose-free formula at 150 cc/kg/day
- Replacement: ORS 10 ml/kg for each diarrhea stool

MODERATE DEHYDRATION: 6% TO 10%

- Rehydration: ORS 100 ml/kg over 4 hours
- Maintenance: Resume a lactose free formula at 150 ml/kg/day
- Replacement: ORS 10 ml/kg for each diarrhea stool

ENERGY (CALORIE) REQUIREMENTS

- *Level of energy intake from food that will balance expenditure when the individual has a body size and composition and level of physical activity consistent with long-term good health; and which allow for the maintenance of economically necessary and socially acceptable activity. In children and pregnant or lactating women the energy requirement includes the energy needs associated with the deposition of tissues or secretion of milk at rates consistent with good health.*[7]

1. Energy requirements per kg body weight are highest during the neonatal period and decline progressively until adult age.

Table 5-6

Electrolyte Composition of Oral Rehydration Solutions

	Na	K	Cl	Citrate	Carbohydrate
		mEq/L			g/L
Oral rehydration solution (ORS) WHO	90	20	80	30	20 (Glucose)
Rehydralyte (rehydration solution) (Ross, Columbus, Ohio)	75	20	65	30	25 (Glucose)
EquaLYTE (rehydration solution) (Ross)	78.2	22.3	67.7	30.1	30 (Glucose 20 g * FOS 10 g)
Pedialyte (maintenance solution) (Ross)	45	20	35	30	25 (Glucose)
Infalyte (maintenance solution) (Mead Johnson, Evansville, Ind)	50	25	45	34	30 (Rice-syrup solids)

*FOS: Fructo-oligosaccharide – soluble nondigestable carbohydrates that are rapidly fermented by GI bacteria to produce short-chain fatty acids (SCFA). The SCFA, especially pyruvate, butyrate, and isobutyrate, are preferred fuel for colonocytes. SCFA increase electrolyte and water absorption.[6]

2. Figure 5-2 shows the average caloric requirements throughout childhood. These represent averages only and should be thought of as a place to start. Individual children may require more or less energy depending on many factors, such as activity, body composition, disease state etc.
   A. The low birth weight infant may require 150 kcal/kg while normal birth weight infants require 100 to 120 kcal/kg.
   B. The caloric requirements in healthy non-stressed infants aged birth to 1 year are 100 to 115 kcal/kg/day.

Resting Energy Expenditure

- The components of total daily energy expenditure in children[8] are: 1) basal metabolism (~REE); 2) physical activity; 3) energy cost of growth; 4) thermic effect of food (~5 kcal/kg/d); 5) thermoregulation; and 6) losses (~5 kcal/kg/d).
- Resting energy expenditure (REE) is fairly stable and the largest contributor (~50% to 70%) to daily total energy requirements.
- The total energy requirement is estimated as multiples of REE.

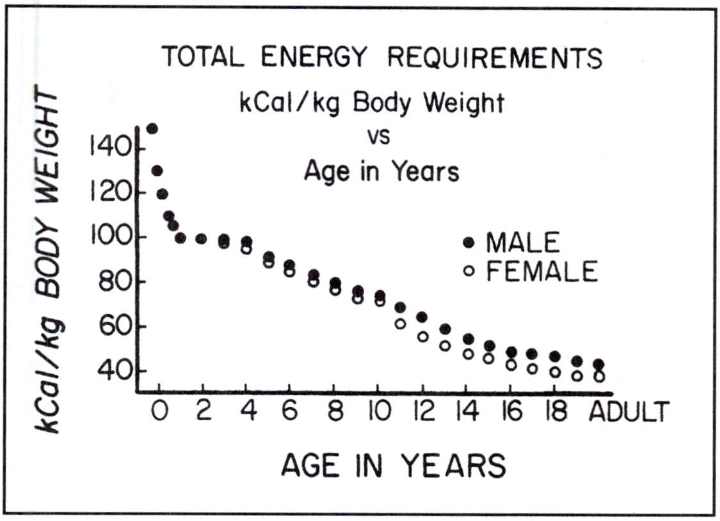

Figure 5-2. Average caloric requirements throughout childhood.

Resting Energy Expenditure, kcal/d Prediction Equations

1. World Health Organization equation (WHO).
2. Schofield equations.
3. Harris Benedict equations.
   - Harris Benedict REE prediction equations are not recommended for use in pediatrics because of having been derived from mostly adult REE measurements.[9]
   - WHO and Schofield REE prediction equations are the most appropriate and widely used in infants, children, and adolescents. Both are very reliable in healthy children aged >1 year.
   - The World Health Organization (WHO) equations predict REE based on age, gender, and weight.[7] See Table 5-7.
   - The Schofield equations[10] predict REE based on age, gender, weight, and length/height. The inclusion of length/height provides for better accuracy when there is altered body composition (eg, children with failure to thrive). See Table 5-8.
   - The predicted REE is multiplied by an activity/stress adjustment factor depending on nutritional status, disease stress, and need or requirement for catch-up growth.[11] See Table 5-9.
   - Reliability and accuracy of prediction equations declines when there is altered body composition (eg, failure to thrive, obesity, and chronic disease). In these situations REE should be measured using indirect calorimetry.[9,12]

Table 5-7

WHO Energy Prediction Equations: REE, kcal/day

Gender	Age, y	REE, kcal/day
Male	1 to 3	60.9W – 54
	3 to 10	22.7W + 495
	10 to 18	17.5W + 651
	18 to 30	15.3W + 679
Female	1 to 3	61W – 51
	3 to 10	22.5W + 499
	10 to 18	12.2W + 746
	18 to 30	14.7W + 496

W = weight, kg

Table 5-8

Schofield Energy Prediction Equations: REE, kcal/day

Gender	Age, y	REE, kcal/day
Male	0 to 3	0.167W + 1517.4H – 617.6
	3 to 10	19.59W + 1303H + 414.9
	10 to 18	16.25W + 137.2H – 515.5
Female	0 to 3	16.252W + 1023.2H – 413.5
	3 to 10	16.969W + 161.8H + 371.2
	10 to 18	8.365W + 465H + 200

W = weight (kg); H = length/height (m)

Example

Estimation of total energy requirements (TEE) of a 4-year-old male toddler, with moderate sepsis in the ICU and previously good nutritional status, body weight 18.5 kg:
Total energy requirements = REE x Activity/Stress factor
REE based on WHO equation: (22.7 x 18.5) + 495 = 915 kcal/day
Estimated stress factor = 1.5
TEE = 915 x 1.5 = 1373 kcal/d

Indirect Calorimetry

- Whenever possible energy requirements should be measured,[7] especially in settings where reliability of prediction equations is limited (eg, during chronic illness, impaired growth [failure to thrive and obesity], altered body composition, and poor response to initial nutritional intervention).

Table 5-9

Activity/Stress Adjustment Factors

REE x 1.3	For a well-nourished child at bed rest with mild to moderate stress (minor surgery)
REE x 1.5	For a normally active child with mild to moderate stress; an inactive child with severe stress (trauma, sepsis, cancer, extensive surgery); or a child with minimal activity and malnutrition requiring catch-up growth
REE x 1.7	For active child requiring catch-up growth or an active child with severe stress

- REE measurement is conducted preferably in the early morning after an age-appropriate fast: 3 to 6 hours in infants, and 8 hours in older children. It is recommended that the measurement last 40 to 60 minutes to allow for adequate equilibration and appropriate editing of the collected data.[13] In order to achieve cooperation and minimize spontaneous movement during REE measurements, younger children may be sedated with a short acting sedative (eg, orally administered chloral hydrate 50 to 65 mg/kg ~30 minutes prior to the test).[12] See more details about indirect calorimetry in Chapter 1.

Interpretation of Measured Resting Energy Expenditure in Children[12-14]

- See Chapter 1 for factors affecting REE measurement.
- Measured REE (REE_M) (kcal/d) is compared with predicted REE (REE_P, kcal/d) using WHO and/or Schofield equations to determine normal or increased metabolic rate as follows:
  - Normal metabolic rate: $REE_M = REE_P$ x (90 to 110%) in subjects without sedation
    $REE_M = REE_P$ x (80 to 100%) in sedated subjects
  - Increased metabolic rate: $REE_M > REE_P$ x 110%
  - Decreased metabolic rate: $REE_M < REE_P$ x 90% in subjects without sedation
    $REE_M < REE_P$ x 80% in seated subjects

Protein Requirements

- *Lowest level of dietary protein intake that will balance the losses of nitrogen from the body in persons maintaining energy balance at modest levels of physical activity. In children and pregnant or lactating women, the protein requirement is taken to include the needs associated with the deposition of tissues or the secretion of milk at rates consistent with good health.*[7]

Figure 5-3. Minimum safe levels of protein intake in children.

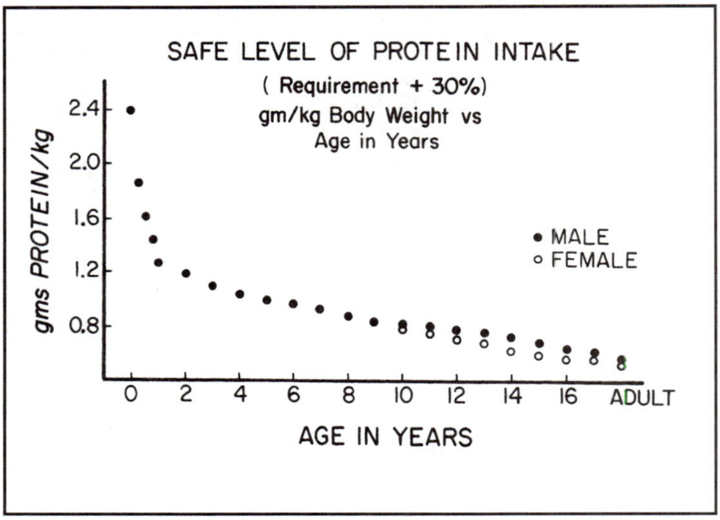

- Protein requirements per kg body weight correlate with a child's rate of growth and are highest at birth and during the first year of life.
- Figure 5-3 shows the minimal protein intake in children. Intakes up to 2 times that shown in the figure can be given safely. Excess protein intakes (>4 g/kg/day) may be accompanied by elevations in BUN, which facilitates urea excretion, and by an increase in urinary calcium. Low birth weight infants fed very high levels of protein (5 to 6g/kg per day) may experience reduced growth rate, urine abnormalities, lethargy, fever, and impairment in neurological development.
- Pre-term infants may be started at 1g/kg/day and advanced by 0.5 to 1 g/kg/day up to a maximum of 3.0 to 3.5 g/kg/day. Children 1 to 12 months old require 2.0 to 3.0 g/kg/day; 1.5 to 2.5 g/kg/day for children 1 to 8 years old, and 0.8 to 1.5 g/kg/day after age 8 years.

Electrolytes, Vitamins, Minerals, and Trace Elements

Appendix A, Tables 10 through 13 show the guidelines for the use of vitamins, electrolytes and mineral supplements in healthy infants and children. Children that might benefit from supplements include: those with feeding problems and picky eating behaviors, those recovering from malnutrition, those with gastrointestinal disorders associated with malabsorption, and those with metabolic disorders or medical therapy requiring restricted diets. Intravenous vitamin recommendations are found in Appendix A, Table 26.

- Fetal accretion of calcium and phosphorus are approximately 130 mg/kg/day and 75 mg/kg/day respectively.
- Generally iron supplementation is unnecessary in healthy term infants aged <2 months. However, because most fetal iron accretion occurs during the last

trimester, preterm infants are at risk of iron deficiency and therefore should be supplemented 200 mg/kg/day. Exclusively breast fed infants may also be at risk of inadequate iron intake and therefore should receive 100 mg/kg/day.

Parenteral Nutrition

Indications

Parenteral nutrition is used whenever there is failure or inability of adequate nutritional support through the gastrointestinal tract because of developmental, medical, or surgical reasons. Conditions commonly necessitating parenteral nutrition support include extreme prematurity with its medical and surgical complications, short bowel syndrome (may result from congenital intestinal atresia, volvulus, intussusception, gastroschisis, omphalocele, necrotizing enterocolitis, vascular infarction, and small bowel aganglionosis related to Hirschsprung's Disease). Parenteral nutrition may also be required in infants, children and adolescents requiring brief or prolonged nutrition support (eg, during critical illness, illnesses with severe small intestinal mucosal damage related to protein intolerance or infection, chemotherapy, gastrointestinal surgery, and chronic intestinal pseudo-obstruction syndromes).

- Parental nutrition is frequently used during nutritional support of preterm[15] infants with difficulty tolerating enteral feeding during the first few days or weeks after birth. Parenteral nutrition may also serve to supplement enteral feedings, which are being slowly advanced.

Peripheral Parenteral Nutrition

Dextrose concentrations ≤12.5% and 2% amino acids.

- Starting volume should meet maintenance fluid requirements.
- For premature infants, increase over 12 to 24 hours to reach the desired rate of infusion (Table 5-10). The recommended caloric distribution of 8% to 15% protein, 50% to 55% carbohydrate and rest from IV fat emulsion.
- In premature infants, optimal caloric intake may be difficult to reach due to fluid restrictions (approximately 130 ml/kg/day).
- Parenteral nutrition solutions are hyperosmolar with potential for caustic skin infiltrates. Therefore only central veins should be used during infusion of solutions with dextrose concentrations >12.5%.
- X-ray confirmation that the intravenous catheter is positioned in a central vein should be always be obtained prior to infusion of hyperosmolar parenteral nutrition.
- Recommended solutions are shown in Appendix A, Table 31.

Central Parenteral Nutrition

Dextrose concentrations >12.5%

- Start with peripheral strength PN using above guidelines.

TABLE 5-10

Recommended Parenteral Energy Intakes

Weight	Energy (kcal/kg/day)
3 to 12	90 to 110
12 to 25	85 to 90
25 to 35	70 to 80
35 to 50	50 to 65
>50	40

- Advance glucose concentration every 24 hours up to a maximum of 25%. For infants less than 3 months, glucose concentration should be advanced by 2.5% every 24 hours. Glucose should be monitored via serum or urine checks at least daily.
- See Adult Section for catheter care and management guidelines.
- Solutions recommended are shown on Appendix A, Table 32.
- Physical and occupational therapy are recommended to maintain oral motor development and feeding skills especially when prolonged PN (>2weeks) is being used.

COMPONENTS OF PARENTERAL NUTRITION SOLUTIONS

Calories

Patients with critical illness, malnutrition, and need for catch-up growth require additional calories, and those with fluid losses or retention require adjustments in PN fluid and mineral intake.

CALCULATIONS FOR DESIRED RATE OF INFUSION

1. Determine kcal per ml of PN solution and kcal per ml of the fat solution to be used (Appendix A, Table 20) and the kcal per kg needed (Appendix A, Table 21).
2. Approximately 70% of calories to be supplied by the dextrose and amino acids solution:

(Kcal/kg/day x 0.7 = calories per kg supplied by TPN)

3. Approximately 30% of calories to be supplied by the IV fat emulsion solution:

(Kcal/kg/day x 0.3 = calories per kg supplied by fat)

4. Infusion rates:

kg x (kcal/kg x 0.7) divided by 24 hrs = TPN solution, ml per hr TPN solution (kcal/ml)
kg x (kcal/kg x 0.3) divided by 24 hrs = fat solution, ml per hr fat solution (kcal/ml)

Protein (Amino Acids)

- Cysteine may be added to neonate/infant TPN solutions at a dose of 40 mg/g amino acid to increase the solubility of calcium and phosphorus. Cysteine may be essential in premature infants because of the absence of cysthathionase enzyme activity, which converts methionine to cysteine.[16,17] Addition of cysteine also improves nitrogen retention.
- Taurine is contained in the neonatal amino acid solution (trophamine). It is an essential amino acid in these patients because of the delayed cystathionase and cysteine sulfinic acid decarboxylase maturation. Taurine deficiency may lead to retinal abnormalities.
- PN solutions for neonates contain additional tyrosine and histidine because of the limited synthetic capacity for these amino acids in the neonate.
- Neonatal PN amino acid solutions contain a lower phenylalanine concentration because an excessive dose of this amino acid is associated with neurotoxicity in preterm infants.
- Amino acid solutions for pediatric use are based on the concentration necessary to maintain a plasma amino acid profile similar to breast milk.
- Carnitine facilitates transport of fatty acids into the mitochondria for oxidation. There are conflicting studies about its benefit. Consider supplementation of TPN with carnitine for the extremely low birth weight premature infants, children on long-term TPN therapy, and hypertriglyceridemia. The recommended dose is 10 to 20 mg/kg/day.

IV Fat Emulsion

- Optimally, fat should provide 30% to 40% of total caloric intake, and not to exceed 60% of the total daily calorie intake.
- IV fat emulsion can be started simultaneously with the dextrose/amino acid PN solution, except during the first week of life when IV fat emulsion is usually initiated 2 to 3 days after dextrose amino acid solutions.

- Essential fatty acid deficiency may develop within 1 to 2 days in pre-term infants on PN therapy without lipids because of their limited fat stores.
- Begin with a 20% solution at 5ml/kg/day which equals 1 g/kg/day or 10 kcal/kg/day and initially administer by continuous infusion over 24 hours.
- Check daily serum triglyceride level and if within normal, increase lipid using rate of 0.5 g/kg/day to goal of 3 g/kg, not to exceed 100 g/day.
- Pre-term infants may have a decreased ability to clear the lipid emulsion from the blood stream and therefore, initiation should begin 0.5 g/kg/day and be increased by 0.25 to 0.5 g/kg/day. Rate should not exceed 0.15 g/kg/hr. Lipid emulsions may also increase the risk of kernicterus in jaundiced neonates because the free fatty acids released during hydrolysis of the lipid compete with bilirubin for albumin binding.
- Serum triglycerides should be monitored with very change in lipid infusion.

Electrolytes

- IV electrolyte requirements are found in Appendix A, Table 10.
- Acid-base abnormalities may be corrected with Na or K acetate. It is usually never given at concentrations greater than 3 mmol/dL. Acetate, a bicarbonate precursor, is soluble and stable in parenteral nutrition solutions. Sodium bicarbonate is contraindicated because it will result in calcium/phosphorous precipitation, and also high sodium load.
- Potassium or sodium phosphate may be used to provide phosphorus.
- Calcium/phosphorus solubility in PN solutions depends on pH, temperature, amino acid concentration and the amino acid mixture used. The PN dietitian or pharmacist should be contacted regarding the compatibility of calcium and phosphorus concentrations if they differ from the standard TPN protocol.

Vitamins

- Preterm Infants and neonates <2.5 kg receive MVI-Pediatric 2 ml/kg/day.
- Infants >2.5 kg to 11 yrs: 1 vial (5 ml) MVI-Pediatrics per day.
  MVI-Pediatric contains vitamin K; additional supplementation is unnecessary.
- Adolescents: 1 vial (10 ml) MVI-12 + vitamin K 200 mg per day.
- Concentration of individual vitamins in standard vitamin preparations are shown in Appendix A, Table 26.

Minerals and Trace Elements

- The pharmacy should add the appropriate amounts to meet recommendations shown in Table 5-11.
- Patients with gastrointestinal losses, renal failure, or other special situations may have different requirements to be determined based on underlying disease and serum levels.
- Iron will need to be provided if the patient is NPO longer than 2 months or enteral intake does not meet requirements. However, because of solution

incompatibility, iron dextran and intralipid must be infused from separate bags. Also caution to monitor for iron levels because of increased risk for iron overload associated with long-term PN with iron. Iron in PN therapy may also be associated with increased risk for bacterial sepsis therefore enteral route is always preferred.

Additives

- Insulin may be added to control blood glucose. Use 0.5 to 2.0 units of regular insulin per 10 grams of dextrose.
- Heparin (1 unit/ml) can be added to the solution to reduce the incidence of thrombophlebitis and preserve the patency of the line.
- Medication compatibility with PN is shown in Appendix A, Tables 28 and 29.
- The use of the PN central line for medication is to be discouraged if alternate IVs are available.

Glucose, Amino Acid, and Fat Admixtures

- The dextrose/amino acid PN solution can be combined in one bag with IV fat emulsion to form a 3 in 1 admixture.
- These solutions should only be used in patients whose TPN requirements are stable. They are mostly used in patients on home TPN therapy.
- Because of potential solution instability, never alter the components or concentrations without checking with the nutritional support team or pharmacy.
- Recommendations are shown in Appendix A, Table 33.

Writing Orders

See Figure 5-4.

Monitoring Parenteral Nutrition

Complications of Parenteral Nutrition

See Adult Section and Table 5-12.

Home PN

Also see Adult Section.

The goals of home PN therapy in children should be sustenance of normal growth, definite steps toward intestinal rehabilitation, and prevention of metabolic complications from PN therapy. Successful home PN therapy requires a dedicated multidisciplinary nutrition support team comprised of physician nutritionist, dietician, nurse, pharmacist, surgeon and interventional radiologist. Every child on long-

Table 5-11

Electrolyte and Trace Element Requirements

	Ca (mg/dL)	Mg (mg/L)	P (mg/L)		Zn	Cu	Cr	Mn	Se
Preterm Infants	500-600	50-70	400-450	Infants < 2.5kg (mg/kg/d)	400	40	0.4	10	2
Term Infants	500-600	50-70	400-450	Infants >2.5kg (mg/kg/d)	100	10	0.1	2.5	1.5
Children	200-400	20-40	150-300	Adolescents (mg per day)	4000	1600	16	400	80

CHILDREN'S HOSPITAL, NORTHWESTERN
PEDIATRIC PARENTERAL NUTRITION FORM
Physician Order Form

Date of birth:

Date/Time ____________ Weight ________ kg | Central/PICC | Peripheral | TPN Day # ______

Continue Yesterday's Order
(Any change requires a complete new order)

Volume: _____ mL/day = _____ mL/hr x _____ hrs
____ Hr Cycle: _____ mL/hr x _____ hrs; Ramps: _____ mL/hr x _____ hrs

Specify Macronutrients

Dextrose: ______ % (g/100 mL) Peripheral: ≤ 10% Central: 10 – 20%	Aminoacids: _______g/kg/d (1 – 3g/kg/d)	Aminosyn 10%; Trophamine 10% Novamine 10%; Hepatasol 10% (Select one)

Specify Electrolytes and Micronutrients (Check one) **Standard Electrolytes with MVI**

Sodium acetate _____ mEq/kg/day
Sodium chloride _____ mEq/kg/day
Sodium phosphate _____ mEq/kg/day
(1 mEq Na^+ phosphate = 0.75 mM phosphate)

Total Sodium ______ mEq/kg/day

Potassium acetate _____ mEq/kg/day
Potassium chloride _____ mEq/kg/day
Potassium phosphate _____ mEq/kg/day
(1 mEq K^+ phosphate = 0.68 mM phosphate)

Total Potassium _____ mEq/kg/day

Calcium gluconate
< 10 kg _____ mg/kg/day
> 10 kg _____ mg/day

Magnesium sulfate _____ mEq/kg/day

Trace Elements
(Check one)
Pediatric Trace 0.2 mL/kg/day
(< 50 kg)
Adult Trace (MTE-4) 1 mL/day
(> 50 kg)

Pediatric MVI
< 1 kg 1.67 mL/day
1 –3 kg 3.25 mL/day
> 3 kg 5 mL/day

Adult MVI-12*(see additional additives)
> 50 kg 10 mL/day

Standard Electrolyte Package
(Check one)

< 50 kg
Na^+ chloride 2 mEq Na^+/kg/day
K^+ phosphate 2 mEq K^+/kg/day
Ca^{++} gluconate
< 10 kg = 100 mg/kg/day
> 10 kg = 1000 mg/day
Magnesium 0.3 mEq/kg/day

≥ 50 kg
Na^+ chloride 1 mEq Na^+/kg/day
K^+ phosphate 1 mEq K^+/kg/day
Ca^{++} gluconate 1000 mg/day
Magnesium 0.3 mEq/kg/day

Normal Daily Requirements
Sodium 2-4 mEq/kg
Potassium 1-2 mEq/kg
Chloride 2-4 mEq/kg
Calcium 100-400 mg/kg
Phosphorus 0.5-1 mM/kg
Magnesium 0.2-0.5 mEq/kg

Specify Additional Additives

Heparin 1 unit/mL (Central/PICC access) ______________________

Ranitidine ______ mg/kg/day (1-2 mg/kg/day) ______________________

*Vitamin K 10 mg Q ________ if receiving MVI-12 ______________________
(Once a week) ______________________

Specify Lipids

_____ g/kg/day x _____ (weight, kg) x 5 mL = _____ mL/day
20% Lipids: infusion rate = _______ mL/hr x _______ hr

See reverse side for guidelines. Physician ________________ Date/Time ________

Figure 5-4. Sample TPN lipid order form.

ℹ **Initial orders must be submitted to Pharmacy by 3:30 PM.**

Guidelines for Pediatric Parenteral Nutrition (PN)

Initiation and Advancement of Macronutrients*

Initiation	
Dextrose	10% to 12.5%
Protein	1-1.5 g/kg/day
Lipids	0.5 g/kg/day
Advancement	
Dextrose	2.5% to 5% Increments per day
Protein	0.5 g/kg/day
Lipids	0.5 g/kg/day
Maximum	
Dextrose	30%
Protein	3.5 g/kg/day
Lipids	3 g/kg/day

Protein Source

Aminosyn, a crystalline amino acid mixture of essential and nonessential amino acids. Has higher ratio of essential to nonessential amino acids.

Trophamine, provided for patients aged ≤ 6-months. Composed of essential and nonessential L-aminoacids in a pattern appropriate for normal growth in infants

Novamine, provided for patients aged ≥ 6-months. Composed of essential and nonessential L-aminoacids in a pattern appropriate for normal growth in children

Hepatasol, enriched in branched amino acids (isoleucine, leucine, valine) and has reduced amounts of methionine and aromatic amino acids (phenylalanine, tryptophan, tyrosine). It is available for patients with severe liver failure and hepatic encephalopathy. (However, data supporting use is inconclusive)

Recommended Laboratory Monitoring

	Baseline	Daily Until Stable	Weekly	Monthly
Na, K, Cl, CO_2	X	X	X	
Glucose, BUN, Cr	X	X	X	
Ionized Ca	X	X	X	
Phos, Mg	X	X	X	
Triglycerides		Day #3	X	X
AST, Alk Phos	X		X	X
GGT	X			X
Prealbumin	X			
Bilirubin (T/D)	X			

Composition of Trace Elements (per 1 mL)

	Pedtrace®-4	M.T.E.®-4
Chromium	1 mcg	10 mcg
Copper	0.1 mg	1 mg
Manganese	0.03 mg	0.5 mg
Zinc	0.5 mg	5 mg

- Severe liver disease, eliminate copper and manganese.
- Severe renal disease, eliminate selenium, chromium, zinc

Additional Micronutrients Required In Prolonged (> 4-6 weeks) TPN

Selenium 3 mcg/kg/day

Calculations

Dextrose: $\dfrac{\_\_\_\_\text{ g X }\_\_\_\_\text{ mL/day}}{100\text{ mL}} = \_\_\_\_\text{ g/day}$

$\dfrac{\_\_\_\_\text{ g}}{\text{Wt (kg) x 1.44}} = \_\_\_\_\text{ mg/kg/min}$

Protein: $\dfrac{\_\_\_\_\text{ g X }\_\_\_\_\text{ mL/day}}{100\text{ mL}} = \_\_\_\_\text{ g/day}$

Nitrogen: _____ g protein/day ÷ 6.25 = _____ g N/day

Fat: _____ mL/day X 0.2 g/mL = _____ g/day

Calorie Count

Dextrose: _____ g/day X 3.4 Kcal/g = _____ Kcal/day

Protein: _____ g/day X 4 Kcal/g = _____ Kcal/day

Fat: _____ mL 20% lipid/day X 2 Kcal/mL = _____ Kcal/day

Non-protein Calorie Count : Nitrogen (150-200 NPC:N)

$\dfrac{(\_\_\_\_\text{ Kcal/day dextrose + }\_\_\_\_\text{ Kcal/day fat})}{\_\_\_\_\text{ g Nitrogen/day}}$

Composition of Multiple Vitamins

	M.V.I.® Pediatric per vial (5 mL)	M.V.I.® -12 (vial 1+2 10 mL)
Vitamin A (retinol)	2300 units	3300 units
Vitamin D (ergocalciferol)	400 units	200 units
Vitamin E (tocopherol)	7 units	10 units
Vitamin B_1 (thiamine)	1.2 mg	3 mg
Vitamin B_2 (riboflavin)	1.4 mg	3.6 mg
Vitamin B_3 (niacinamide)	17 mg	40 mg
Vitamin B_5 (dexpanthenol)	5 mg	15 mg
Vitamin B_6 (pyridoxine)	1 mg	4 mg
Vitamin B_{12} (cyanocobalamin)	1 mcg	5 mcg
Vitamin C (ascorbic acid)	80 mg	100 mg
Biotin	20 mcg	60 mcg
Folic acid	0.14 mg	0.4 mg
Vitamin K (phytonadione)	200 mcg	NONE

* Rate of advancement may be limited by metabolic tolerance (e.g., hyperglycemia, azotemia, hypertriglyceridemia)

Figure 5-4 continued. Sample TPN lipid order form.

Table 5-12

Parenteral Nutrition Monitoring Parameters

	Neonates		Beyond Neonatal Period	
	First Week	**After First Week**	**First Week**	**After First Week**
Strict I&O	Daily	Daily	Daily	Daily
Urine Glucose	q void	q shift	q void	q shift
Electrolytes, BUN	2 to 3 x week	q week	2-3 x week	q week
Ca, PO4, Mg, bili, Alt	q week	q 2 week	q week	q 2 week
Alk phos, albumin	—	q 2 week	q week	q 2 week
Prealbumin	—	As needed	—	As needed
Serum triglycerides (TG)	See below	See below	See below	See below
Serum Fe, Ferritin, TIBC	—	q 4 week	—	q 4 week

Prealbumin has a half-life of 2 days reflecting acute changes in protein intake; use to monitor the short-term adequacy of protein intake. Serum TG: 4 hours after IV fat emulsion begun and with every increase in rate. Decrease rate if triglyceride >150 mg/dL. Endogenous TG may be elevated during stress so pre-infusion levels are suggested.

term PN therapy should be periodically reviewed to assess whether the goals of PN therapy are being accomplished and decide other medical or surgical intervention will promote intestinal rehabilitation.

1. Cycle the TPN to goal of 10 to 18 hours depending on age, underlying disease, and presence or absence of oral/enteral feeds. Shorter TPN cycles (<12 hours) are more safely administered in older children. Caution in infants (aged <6 to 12 months) because of greater risk for hypoglycemia, glucose intolerance, fluid overload and marginal renal function.
2. Prior to discharge:
   A. Caretaker should meet with nutrition support team members and be given follow-up and contact information to the key team members.
   B. Notify home health care agency 5 days before discharge.
   C. Arrange appropriate follow up appointments for 1 to 2 weeks post discharge.
   D. Make arrangements for school if appropriate.
   E. Notify occupational therapy for instructions regarding oral stimulation and feeding skills if needed.
3. Appendix A, Table 34 shows standard solutions for home use
4. Laboratory monitoring:
   A. If the patient's blood volume is adequate, obtain a Chem 20 and CBC weekly or every 2 weeks until stable; then thereafter every 3 to 4 weeks.
   B. If a Chem 20 is not available, obtain electrolytes weekly or every 2 weeks until stable, then thereafter every 3 to 4 weeks.
   C. Iron studies and reticulocyte count every 4 weeks, especially if no iron in TPN.
   D. If indication for TPN therapy includes nutritional rehabilitation, monitor serum pre-albumin every 2 to 4 weeks.
   E. These recommendations are guidelines and may need to be individualized.
5. Daily monitoring:
   A. Temperature daily. Urine glucose twice daily for at least 1 week especially after a TPN change.
   B. All febrile illnesses (38.5°C) must be immediately evaluated with blood and urine cultures, and empirically treated with appropriate IV antibiotics for 48 hr for rule out sepsis. If microbial cultures are positive, antibiotic coverage should be adjusted to sensitivity pattern. Fungal infections require removal of central line.
6. Nutritional assessment during home TPN therapy:
   A. Dietary analysis to evaluate the adequacy of nutrient intake monthly includes enteral intake, iron, and micronutrients.
   B. Infant's (age birth to 6 months) length, weight and head circumference should be monitored and plotted on the appropriate growth charts every 2 weeks.
   C. Older children (age >6 months) should have weight, length/height and head circumference should be checked at least monthly.
   D. Older children who are stable on long-term home TPN therapy should have growth, nutritional status, and labs evaluated no less frequently than trimonthly intervals.

Enteral Nutrition

Transition to Enteral Feeding

- Neonates need to be weaned slowly over 1 to 2 days.
- When stopped, ensure that essential fatty acid needs are met enterally (4% of total calories).

Feeding Methods

Nipple Feeding

- Breast or bottle
- Attempt with infants that are at least 32 weeks of gestation age.

Preterm Infants[18]

- Initial enteral tube feeds are used in infants with birth weight <1.5 kg. Choice between orogastric vs. nasogastric route appears to be of little clinical importance. However, orogastric route should be considered in small pre-term infants who are obligatory nose breathers.
- Non-nutritive sucking should be encouraged when enteral feeds are being used.
- Breast milk is the first-choice milk for preterm infant and preterm formula is second choice.
- Feeds should not be increased more than 24 to 30 ml/kg/day because rapid increase may raise the risk of necrotizing enterocolitis.
- In infants unable to tolerate enteral nutrition trophic feeds ~12 to 24 ml/kg/day should be introduced except where contraindicated.
- Breast milk fortifier is preferably introduced once infants are tolerating ≥90 ml/kg/day of expressed breast milk.
- Ultimately there is very little difference in toleration of feeds between continuous versus bolus feeds. If difficulties occur with one approach then change to the other.
- Nocturnal continuous infusion is important for preventing hypoglycemia in children with glycogen storage disease.
- Weight gain goals for preterm infants are 15 to 20 g/kg/day.

Human Milk

- Human milk contains approximately 20 kcal/oz (0.67 calories per ml). Enfamil Human Milk Fortifier (Mead Johnson, Evansville, Ind) may be used to increase the caloric density, protein and mineral content of human milk for low birth weight infants.
- Initiation of fortifier is recommended after infants are tolerating 90 cc/kg/day of expressed breast milk. When initiating fortification in low birth weight infants, start with 2 packets per 100 cc for the first day (22 kcal/oz) and increase to 4 packets per 100 cc (24 kcal/oz) on the second day. Do not add fortifier to breast milk in a ratio greater than 1 packet per 25 cc. See Appendix C, Table 5 for details about fortifiers.

- Special concerns when feeding human milk by gavage: The use of continuous drip with human milk may result in substantial losses of fat unless an automatic syringe pump is used and the tip of the syringe is oriented upright to avoid loss of fat.
- "Hind milk" is considered an energy supplement due to its high fat content.

Infant Formulas

Breast-feeding is the optimal mode of feeding the normal term infant, but because not all infants have access to human milk, nutritious alternatives to human milk have been developed. The composition of infant formulas has evolved over the past century to provide specific needs depending on nutrient requirements, absorptive physiology, disease state, metabolic disturbances, and goals of nutritional support.

- Standard infant formulas are based on caloric and nutrient composition of breast milk, and generally provide 20 kcal/oz or 0.67 kcal/ml. When additional calories are desired for various reasons (eg, fluid restriction, catch-up growth), the formula can be concentrated (see Table 5-13) or modular products such as lipids, carbohydrates and proteins can be added.
- Concentrating formulas increases the osmolality and likelihood of intolerance. The risk for excessive renal solute load is greatest at concentrations of >27 Kcal/oz in premature babies and young infants. There are higher calorie premixed pre-term infant formulas that may be preferable in these situations and the advantage of increased nutrients with controlled electrolytes and osmolality. See Appendix C, Table 5.

Milk-Based Formulas

Standard milk-protein-based formulas normally used for routine infant feeding. Lacto-free formulations are available when lactose intolerance is suspected or diagnosed, but milk-protein-based formula is desired. Selection of the proper formula requires knowledge of its composition and intended use. The composition of the standard milk-based infant formulas is shown in the formula tables in Appendix C, Table 3.

Soy-Based Formulas

Examples of soy protein-based formulas are: Isomil and Alsoy (Ross, Columbus, Ohio) and Prosobee (Mead Johnson, Evansville, Ind). Composition of soy-based formulas is shown in Appendix C, Table 4. Soy protein-based formulas may be used when there is cow milk protein intolerance; however, cross reactivity may occur in more than half of affected infants. Other indications are when a lactose-free diet is desired (eg, galactosemia, primary lactose intolerance, and secondary lactose intolerance that may complicate severe gastroenteritis). Prosobee may be appropriate when there is suspected sucrase deficiency during transient or chronic diarrhea.

Formulas Designed for Premature and Low Birth Weight Infants

Premature and low birth weight formulas are listed in Appendix C, Table 5. These formulas are specially suited for the immature gastrointestinal tract and are designed to support postnatal growth at intrauterine rates. They differ from standard infant formulas in the following aspects: 1) lower lactose content because of marginal lactase activity in preterm infants and 2) higher protein content because of

TABLE 5-13

Formula Preparation

Concentration	Amount of powder/liquid	Water (oz)
20 kcal/oz (0.67 kcal/ml)	1 cup powdered formula	29
	4 scoops powdered formula	8
	13 oz liquid concentrate	13
24 kcal/oz (0.8 kcal/ml)	1 cup powdered formula	24
	5 scoops powdered formula	8
	13 oz liquid concentrate	9
27 kcal/oz (0.9 kcal/ml)	1 cup powdered formula	21
	5.5 scoops powdered formula	8
	13 oz liquid concentrate	6
30 kcal/oz (1.0 kcal/ml)	1 cup powdered formula	18
	6 scoops powdered formula	8
	13 oz liquid concentrate	4

1 scoop = 1 measuring table spoon

greater protein (g/kg) requirements in preterm infants. The protein is provided in a similar ratio (whey: caseine; 60:40) as breast milk so that postprandial plasma amino acid profiles resemble those of breast milk. 3) Fat content is made up of 40% to 50% medium chain triglycerides (MCT) because of the post-conceptual delay in pancreatic enzyme activity. The long chain triglycerides (LCTs) are enriched with essential fatty acids. 4) Increased calcium and phosphorous supports optimal bone mineralization. 5) Increased caloric density supports optimal growth rates.

Specialized Formulas

Specialized infant formulas are listed in Appendix C, Table 6. These formulas are not indicated for use in the normal infant. They include protein hydrolysate and elemental formulas indicated for cow/soy-protein intolerance and severe or multiple food allergies; MCT enriched formulas for malabsorption disorders—eg, pancreatic insufficiency, cholestasis, biliary obstruction, lymphangiectasia.

Nutritionals

These formulas are designed to meet the recommended dietary allowances (RDA) for children aged 1 to 10 years in less volume than adult formulas. Several adult enteral products can also be used for the pediatric patient older than 1 year of age; however, they have a higher protein and sodium content, higher vitamin/mineral base and unless otherwise indicated, and most require administration by enteral tube because of poor palatability. Most provide 1 kcal/ml. However the products vary in osmolality, protein source, MCT: LCT ratio, and caloric density. Newer formulas are supplemented with certain disease modulating nutrients—eg, glutamine, omega fatty acids and transforming growth factor beta (TGF-β). See Appendix C, Tables 7 and 8.

Modular Formulas

The products were developed to help treat specific nutritional problems. They are not complete diets and care should be taken to make sure the patient's total intake is adequate when using them. They include Ross Carbohydrate Free (RCF) (Ross, Columbus, Ohio) formula and Product 3232 A (Ross), which may be used during management of various forms of carbohydrate intolerance (eg, intractable diarrhea, glycogen storage disease, and hereditary fructose intolerance). Product 80056 A (Mead Johnson, Evansville, Ind) and ProVimin (Ross). They are listed with the specialized formulas. See Appendix C, Table 9.

Infant Formula Additives

Many nutrients are available to increase specific nutrient or calorie concentrations in infant formulas. These for both cow and goat milk are listed in Appendix C, Table 10.

Special Metabolic Formulas and Modules

Special formulas designed for source in various metabolic disorders including inborn errors in amino acid metabolism where dietary control of specific nutrients is necessary. These are listed in Appendix C, Tables 11 to 13.

Transition to Solid Food

Because iron stores are limited in the infant, the first solid food recommended is iron-fortified infant cereal. After this, the sequence of introduction is dictated primarily by tradition and is listed in the following table:

Month	*Food Items*
1-4	Breast milk or formula only
4-6	Iron-fortified cereal
6-7	Strained fruits; begin introducing cup
7-8	Strained vegetables
8-9	Start finger foods and chopped (junior food)
9	Meats, citrus juice
10	Bite-sized cooked foods
12	All table foods

Complications of Enteral Feeding

See Adult Section.

References

1. Zemel BS, Riley EM, Stallings VA. Evaluation of methodology for nutritional assessment in children: anthropometry, body composition, and energy expenditure. *Annu Rev Nutr.* 1997;17:211-35.
2. Kerr DS. Failure to thrive and malnutrition. In Kleigman RM, Nieder ML, Super DM (eds). *Practical Strategies in Pediatric Diagnosis and Therapy.* Philadelphia: WB Saunders; 1996;243-57.
3. Holliday MA, Segar WE. The maintenance need for water in parenteral fluid therapy. *Pediatrics.* 1957;19:823-32.
4. Holliday MA, Segar WE. Reducing errors in fluid therapy management. *Pediatrics.* 2003;111(2):424-5.
5. Duggan C, Santosham M, Glass RI. The management of acute diarrhea in children: Oral rehydration, maintenance and nutritional therapy. *MMWR.* 1992;41:1-20.
6. Royall D, Wolever TMS, Jeejeebhoy KN. Clinical significance of colonic fermentation. *Am J Gastroenterol.* 1990;85:1307-12.
7. World Health Organization. *Energy and protein requirements. Report of a joint FAO/WHO/UNU Expert Consultation.* (WHO Technical Report Series No. 724). Geneva: World Health Organization; 1985.
8. Wells JCK, Davies PSW. The components of energy metabolism in 12-week infants. *Annals of Human Biology.* 1995;22(2):175-80.
9. Kaplan AS, Zemel BS, Neiswender KM, Stallings VA. Resting energy expenditure in clinical pediatrics: Measured versus prediction equations. *J Pediatr.* 1995;127:200-5.
10. Schofield WN, Schofield C, James WPT. Basal metabolic rate—review and prediction, together with annotated bibliography of source material. *Hum Nutr: Clin Nutr.* 1985;39C (Suppl):5-41.
11. National Academy of Sciences. *Recommended Dietary Allowances.* Washington, DC: National Academy Press; 1989:24-38.
12. Sentongo TA, Tershakovec AM, Mascarenhas MR, Watson MH, Stallings VA. Resting energy expenditure and prediction equations in young children with failure to thrive. *J Pediatr.* 2000;136:345-50.
13. Stallings VA. Resting energy expenditure. In: Altschuler SM, Liacouras CA (eds). *Clinical Pediatric Gastroenterology.* Philadelphia: Churchill Livingstone; 1998; 607-11.
14. Firouzbakhsh S, Mathis RK, Dorchester WL, et al. Measuring resting energy expenditure in children. *J Pediatr Gastroenterol Nutr.* 1993;16:136-42.
15. Thureen PJ, Hay WW. Intravenous nutrition and postnatal growth of the micropremie. *Clin Perinatol.* 2000;27(1):197-219.
16. Sturman A, Gaull G, Raiha NCR. Absence of cystathionese in human fetal liver: Is cystine essential? *Pediatrics.* 1995;19:114-118.
17. Mirtallo JM. Parenteral Formulas. In: Rombeau JL, Rolandelli RH (eds). *Clinical Nutrition. Parenteral Nutrition.* 3rd ed. Philadelphia: WB Saunders; 2001:118-139.
18. Newell SJ. Enteral feeding of the mircopremie. *Clin Perinatol.* 2000;27(1):221-34.

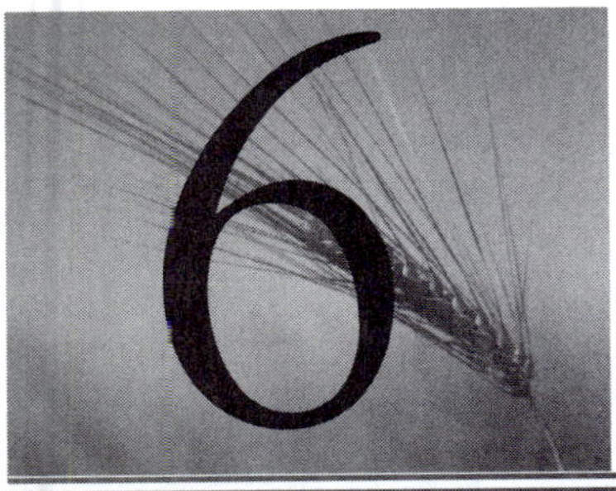

6 Nutritional Support During Pregnancy

Adequate nutrition during pregnancy is mandatory to ensure proper fetal development and maternal health.

- Malnutrition during pregnancy is associated with a high incidence of fetal death, prematurity, low birth weight, and decreased brain size.
- Possible indications for parenteral nutrition during pregnancy include: hyperemesis gravidarum, active Crohn's disease, or disease restricting oral intake, anorexia, cystic fibrosis, pancreatitis.
- See Appendix A, Table 44 for laboratory changes during pregnancy.

Weight Gain

- 10% 1st trimester
- 20% to 30% 2nd trimester; >0.5 to 1.0 lb (0.2 to 0.5 kg) per week
- 60% 3rd trimester
- Total + 20 to 25 (9 to 12 kg) lb
- Weight gain <14 lb (6.5 kg) = weight loss

Targets for Weight Gain

- >120% IBW
    - Total 3 to 4 kg (7 to 8 lb) = 300 g/wk
- IBW (patient not planning to nurse infant)
    - Total 4.5 kg (10 lb) = 350 g/wk
- IBW (will nurse infant)
    - Total 5.5 kg (12 lb) = 400 g/wk
- <90% IBW
    - Total 6.3 to 6.8 kg (14 to 15 lb) = 500 g/wk

Metabolic Changes

These should be anticipated when providing nutritional support:

- Plasma glucose concentration declines
- Stimulated insulin secretion increases
- Peripheral insulin resistance
- Altered lipid metabolism with increased very low-density lipoprotein (VLDL), total cholesterol, low-density lipoprotein (LDL), and high-density lipoprotein (HDL)

Nutritional Requirements

Calories

RDA + 300 kcal/d = 55,000 extra calories for pregnancy

- Recommendation recently questioned[1]
- Lactation: RDA + 525 to 745 kcal/day assuming 600 to 850 ml/day milk produced

Protein

RDA + 10 g/day 1st trimester, add 1.3 g/day

or

1st trimester:	add 1.3 g/day
2nd trimester:	add 6.1 g/day
3rd trimester:	add 10.7 g/day
Lactation:	add 1.5 g/kg/day[2]

Fat

- Extreme dietary deficiency of essential fatty acids is associated with decreased brain lipid content and impaired learning ability in newborn animals
- Monitor the serum triglyceride concentration
- Necessary for prostaglandin synthesis
- An additional 1.5% of total maternal calories should be provided as linoleic acid[3]

Minerals and Trace Elements

- For the RDA of mineral and vitamins during pregnancy and location see Appendix A, Tables 11 through 13
- There is little data on optimal parenteral requirements

CALCIUM, MAGNESIUM

- May decline by 10% to 15% usually related to decreased serum albumin caused by hemodilution

ZINC

- Plasma concentration declines 20% to 25% beginning in the mid 1st trimester
- This may also be related to decreased serum albumin
- Deficiency may cause fetal growth retardation, multiple congenital abnormalities, particularly of the skeletal and nervous systems, and low birth weight

IRON

- Deficiency is associated with infant anemia

COPPER

- Serum concentration increases up to 1.5 to 4x pregnancy, paralleling the increase in ceruloplasmin
- Deficiency (rare) is associated with placental insufficiency and intrauterine death

Vitamins

NIACIN

- Urinary excretion of one metabolite, H-methyl nicotinamide increases during the 2nd trimester

PYRIDOXINE

- Plasma concentration decreases in the 3rd trimester

VITAMIN B_{12}

- Plasma concentration decreases up to 1000 pg/dl throughout pregnancy

FOLATE

- Decrease is most likely related to the depletion of maternal stores
- The greatest risk of deficiency is in multigravida and in mothers receiving anticonvulsants
- Deficiency is associated with fetal neural tube defects, toxemia of pregnancy, and premature labor

ASCORBIC ACID (VITAMIN C)

- Plasma concentration decreases 10% to 15% but is without known consequence, although an association with premature membrane rupture has been reported

THIAMINE

- Urinary thiamine excretion increases during the 2nd and 3rd trimesters
- There is no change in erythrocyte transketolase, however

- Deficiency may cause fatal heart failure in the newborn

RIBOFLAVIN

- Urinary excretion increases during the 2nd trimester and decreases during the 3rd trimester. There is no change in erythrocyte glutathione reductase activity

VITAMIN A

- Serum concentration decreases during the 1st trimester, then gradually increases throughout the remainder of pregnancy
- Megadoses (>8000 IV/day) are associated with congenital urinary tract malformation and neural tube defects

VITAMIN D

- The serum 25-OH D_3 concentration is usually unchanged during pregnancy, but deficiency may be associated with neonatal hypocalcemia and osteomalacia

VITAMIN E

- The serum concentration may increase by 40% to 60% beginning in the 2nd trimester

VITAMIN K

- No increase in the prothrombin time has been observed during pregnancy in the absence of fat malabsorption or bacterial overgrowth

REFERENCES

1. Mughal MM, Shaffer JL, Turner M, et al. Nutritional management of pregnancy in patients on home parenteral nutrition. *Br J Obstet Gynecol.* 1987;94:44-9.
2. Motil KJ, Montandon CM, Thotathuchery M, et al. Dietary protein and nitrogen balance in lactating and nonlactating women. *Am J Clin Nutr.* 1990;51:378-84.
3. Crawford MA. Estimation of essential fatty acid and requirements in pregnancy and lactation. *Prog Food Nutr Sci.* 1980;4:75-80.

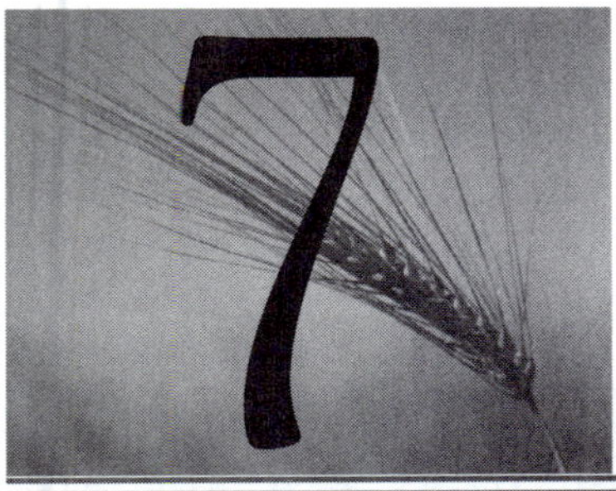

7 Assessing the Efficacy of Nutritional Therapy

Nutritional goals should be established and re-evaluated at regular intervals.

Daily Input and Output Record

Evaluate the input and output record daily to determine what proportion of the prescribed nutritional order is actually received. Interrupted delivery of parenteral nutrition is not uncommon (eg, during blood transfusion). Intravenous pumps may often be 10% and occasionally up to 25% inaccurate. Likewise, enteral nutrition is often interrupted because of medical procedures, tube repositioning, etc.

Weight

Comparison of serial weights is an easy way to assess response to nutritional therapy. If weight gain is anticipated, it should be on the order of 2 to 3 pounds (1 to 2 kg) weekly. Weight gain greater than this, especially during parenteral nutrition, is more often due to fluid retention. Physical examination and close inspection of daily inputs and outputs will help to determine if fluid retention is occurring. Often, presacral edema occurs long before pedal edema, especially in a patient lying prone in bed where the lower back and gluteal regions lie in the most dependent position.

Visceral Proteins

Prealbumin is the preferred visceral protein to assess response to nutritional therapy. It should be checked on the fourth day of therapy. Due to its short half-life (1.9 days), an increase in serum prealbumin should be observed within the first 4 to 7 days. This increase is believed to correlate with increased protein synthesis and anabolism.

Because albumin has a very long half-life (21 days), it will not be responsive to short-term changes in visceral protein status and should not be monitored more often than on a weekly basis unless albumin is exogenously infused to treat hypo-oncotic edema.

Increased serum albumin related to exogenous albumin administration has no relationship to changes in nutritional status.

It may be difficult to normalize serum albumin if ongoing losses occur from severe protein losing enteropathy, wound drainage or exudate, burns, or nephrotic syndrome despite provision of nutritionally adequate therapy.

In markedly hypermetabolic patients, such as those with head trauma or spinal cord injuries, anabolism may not be achievable initially. Therefore, the initial goal should be to limit catabolism.

The role of growth factors such as growth hormone and IGF-1 are under investigation in these situations and should not be used outside of investigational protocols because of their expense, undetermined efficacy, and potential metabolic side effects.

Cellular Immunity

Total lymphocyte count is one of the earliest indicators to show response to nutritional support. However, non-nutritional factors can obviate use of this parameter.

Nitrogen Balance

A negative N balance is associated with catabolism while a positive N balance is associated with net N retention and anabolism. Positive N balance greater than four is desirable.

N balance can be determined after 3 to 4 days of nutritional support to assess the adequacy of caloric and protein provision. A positive N balance requires both sufficient protein and calories.

Physical Examination

Signs of specific nutrient deficiencies and nutritionally dependent processes such as wound healing and fistula closure should be monitored to show improvement and/or resolution.

Muscle Function

Hand grip strength or maximal inspiratory/expiratory pressure can be followed. Skeletal muscle strength can be measured using handgrip dynamometry,[1,2] or maximal inspiratory or expiratory force.[3] Both are excellent methods of assessment, but require patient cooperation, which may be impossible in a physically disabled or ventilated patient, respectively.

Drug-Nutrient Interaction

Certain nutrient deficiencies may occur during treatment despite the provision of a usual maintenance dose of the nutrient in question. See Appendix A, Table 43 for potential drug-nutrient interactions, which may require additional supplementation of some nutrients. Also see Appendix A, Table 45.

References

1. Klidjian AM, Foster KJ, Kammerling RM. Relation of anthropometric and dynamometric variables to serious postoperative complications. *Br Med J.* 1980;281:899-901.
2. Hunt DR, Rowlands BJ, Johnston D. Hand grip strength-a simple prognostic indicator in surgical patients. *JPEN.* 1985;9:701-4.
3. Kelly SM, Rose A, Field S. Inspiratory muscle strength and body composition in patients receiving total parenteral nutrition therapy. *Am Rev Respir Dis.* 1984;130:33-7.

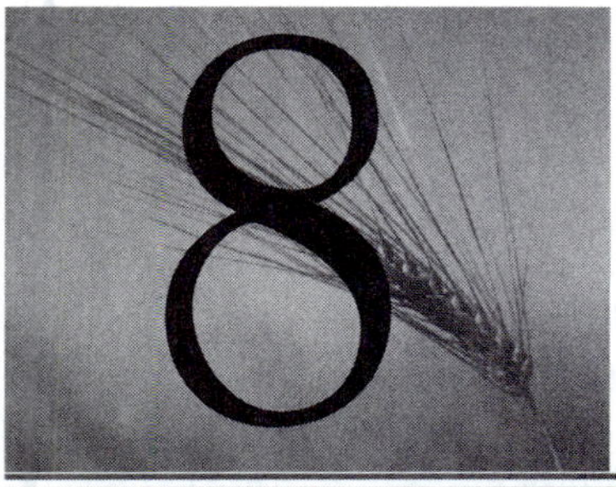

8 Disease-Specific Nutrition

Acute Renal Failure

Restrict protein intake to 0.8 g/kg/day in non-dialyzed patients. Patients fed 0.6 to 0.7 g/kg/day become protein malnourished and have a poorer outcome. There is a theoretical advantage to using formulas containing only essential amino acids, but *no proven clinical efficacy*.[1,2] These formulations are also substantially more expensive than standard amino acid solutions. Provide 35 kcal/day or use indirect calorimetry. Monitor fluid load, serum potassium, and phosphate closely. Renal failure specific formulas such as AminAid (Hormel, Irvine, Calif), Suplena (Ross, Columbus, Ohio), or Nepro (Ross) may be useful in patients with hyperkalemia, hypermagnesemia, or hyperphosphatemia with standard products. However, there is no demonstrated benefit with respect to morbidity or mortality with these products.

Chronic Renal Failure

Protein intake should not be restricted, but increased to account for amino acid loss in the dialysate. This amounts to 6 to 8 g in hemodialysis, 12 to 16 g during peritoneal dialysis, and 12 to 16 g/day for continuous hemofiltration.[3] The amino acid histidine is considered essential in renal failure. Water soluble vitamin deficiency can occur, most especially pyridoxine (B_6) because these vitamins are removed in the dialysate. In contrast, fat soluble vitamins are not removed. Vitamin E is essentially nontoxic and 1,25 dihydroxy-vitamin D concentration is likely to be low on the basis of decreased a-hydroxylation in the kidney. Vitamin A accumulation and toxicity may, however, be a concern. Provide 35 kcal/kg/day or use indirect calorimetry. Patients with chronic renal failure may exhibit fat intolerance and, therefore, the serum triglyceride concentration should be followed carefully to ascertain adequate clearance of lipid emulsion.

Respiratory Failure

Care should be taken to avoid overfeeding. Overfeeding may result in increased CO_2 production, which will impede successful ventilator weaning. Avoiding overfeeding is far more important and much less expensive than specialty pulmonary formulas. Pulmocare (Ross, Columbus, Ohio) provides a greater percentage of calories as lipid than dextrose. Theoretically, its metabolism should produce less CO_2. Clinically, the effects on CO_2 production differ little from standard, higher carbohydrate-containing formulas. The use of Pulmocare should be reserved for the marginal patient only. This is the only product in this category for which published clinical data currently exists. The caloric requirements for a nonventilated patient with chronic obstructive pulmonary disease (COPD) may be difficult to estimate. Unlike nutritionally depleted patients without lung disease who may lose 10% or more of their body weight and who have a measured REE less than predicted, patients with similar degrees of weight loss may have a 10% to 25% increase in REE due to the work of breathing.[4] Failure to provide adequate nutrition will eventually result in a reduction in respiratory muscle strength,[5] hypoxic ventilatory drive,[6] and minute ventilation.[6,7] The margin between underfeeding and overfeeding in this patient group may be small and the use of indirect calorimetry is probably prudent. Patients with marginal respiratory function also should not receive excessive amino acids because high nitrogen intake increases the threshold response to CO_2. The serum phosphate concentration should be monitored specifically, as severe hypophosphatemia may lead to prolonged respiratory failure because of skeletal muscle dysfunction and impaired diaphragm contractility.[8-10] Patients with acute respiratory disease system (ARDS) may experience a transient decrease in PaO_2 during lipid emulsion infusion.[11]

Hepatic Failure

See discussion of branched chain amino acids on page 13.

Short Bowel Syndrome

See Algorithm 8-1. Occurs when there is <200 cm of residual bowel following resection or due to congenital malformations. In adults, those patients at greatest nutritional risk are those with <115 cm of intestine in the absence of a colon or those with <60 cm of intestine in the presence of an intact colon in continuity.

Following massive enterectomy, the first concern is to stabilize the patient hemodynamically and provide adequate fluid management. Once this has been accomplished, TPN should be provided using 25 to 30 kcal/kg/day and 1.5 to 2.0 g/kg/day protein as a goal. Standard enteral formula should be introduced after the first week or week 2 postoperatively, depending upon the patient's overall medical condition, but should be avoided in patients requiring blood pressure support. Medical therapy should be directed at enhancing bowel adaption postoperatively. In addition, fluid and nutrient loss should be controlled in order to minimize the amount of parenteral nutrition required. Patients should be encouraged to eat as much as possible.

There is no proven efficacy of high/low carbohydrate or high/low fat diets in the absence of a colon. Similarly, there is no proven utility of a peptide-based diet. The

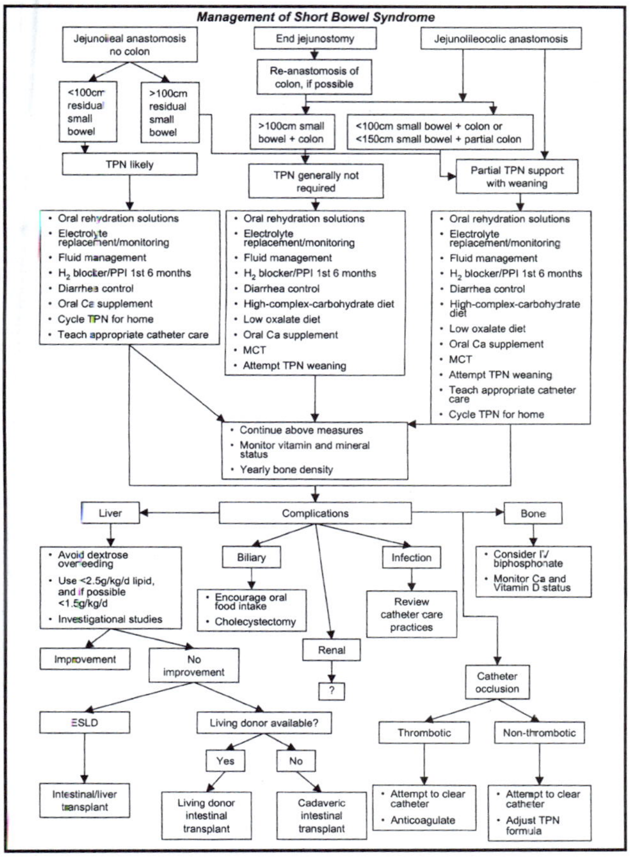

Algorithm 8-1. Short bowel syndrome. (Reprinted from *Gastroenterology*, 124, 4, Buchman AL, et al, AGA technical review on short bowel syndrome and intestinal transplantation, 1111-1134, copyright 2003, with permission from the American Gastroenterological Association.)

colon becomes an important digestive organ via carbohydrate salvage. Unabsorbed soluble fiber and starch that pass into the colon are metabolized by colonic bacterial into short chain fatty acids such as butyrate, the preferred colonocyte fuel. It is theoretically possible to absorb 1000 kcal or more of energy via carbohydrate salvage in a patient with an intact colon. Therefore, a high complex carbohydrate diet with supplemental soluble fiber (oatmeal, oat bran, psyllium, barley, artichokes, strawberries, legumes, prunes, grapefruit, squash) is most appropriate for patients with residual colon in continuity.

MCTs may also serve as a useful caloric source for these patients. Up to 40 to 80 g/day, providing 360 to 720 kcal may be used. MCTs may be used in salad dressing or in baking; it has poor taste alone and smokes at a low temperature and is therefore not a useful general purpose cooking oil.

Oxalate should be restricted in the diet of patients with short bowel syndrome and colon in continuity in order to decrease the risk of development of calcium oxalate nephrolithiasis.

ORS are useful for maintaining intracellular hydration. There are several commercially available solutions or a solution can be made at home by the patient based on the WHO recipe: 1 L tap water, NaCl (2.5 g), KCl (1.5 g), Na_2CO_2 (2.5 g), table sugar (20 g). The optimal sodium content should be 90 to 120 meq/l. If sufficient sodium is available in the diet, ORS are not as critical in the management of patients with colon in continuity.

Transiently (6 months) increased gastric acid secretion occurs following massive small intestinal resection. Therefore, proton pump inhibitors may be useful for

Table 8-1

Vitamin and Mineral Supplements for Patients With Short Bowel Syndrome

Vitamin A	5,000 to 25,000 units daily for correction of deficiency (2,500 for maintenance)
Vitamin B12	1000 mcg subcutaneously monthly for those with terminal ileal resections or disease
Vitamin C	200 to 500 mg daily for replacement (150 mg/d maintenance)
Vitamin D	50,000 units/day for replacement
Vitamin E	400 mg t.i.d for replacement
Vitamin K	10 mg weekly
Calcium	1000 to 2000 mg/day
Magnesium	May require IV replacement
Iron	Iron sulfate (325 mg) or gluconate (300 mg) b.i.d to t.i.d. for replacement
Selenium	60 to 100 ug daily
Zinc	220 to 440 mg daily (sulfate form)
Bicarbonate	As needed

The table lists rough guidelines only. Vitamin and mineral supplementation must be routinely monitored and tailored to the individual patient because relative absorption and requirements may vary.

reducing fluid losses. Fluid losses may also be controlled with anti-motility medications including loperamide hydrochloride and diphenoxylate at doses of 4 to 16 mg daily, Occasionally, especially in patients with end-jejunostomy, codeine sulfate or tincture of opium will be required. Less commonly, octreotide (50 to 100 mg 30 min before meals) may be necessary. Because octreotide may be associated with blunted intestinal adaptation and biliary dysfunction, it should be used only in patients who have >3 L of daily ostomy output despite more conventional treatment. The bile acid sequestering agent cholestyramine is not useful in patients who have had >100 cm of ileum resected because steatorrhea may be increased.

Multiple macronutrient and micronutrient deficiencies may develop. Patients that do not receive full TPN support should receive oral calcium supplements (800 to 1200 mg/day). Magnesium replacement may be problematic because of its cathartic effects, and intravenous replacement may be required. Malabsorption of micronutrients may occur. Fat soluble vitamin deficiency (A, D, E, K) is most common, and should be monitored regularly in patients that do not receive full TPN support. See Table 8-1 for replacement doses. Water soluble vitamin deficiency is less common. Similarly, drug absorption may also be affected and large doses, intravenous, subcutaneous, or sublingual routes may be preferred.

Nutritional Support in Inflammatory Bowel Disease

Macronutrient requirements are similar in patients with either Crohn's disease or ulcerative colitis to the general population, although patients may become malnourished and exhibit protein-calorie malnutrition or specific micronutrient deficiencies because of decreased food intake, malabsorption, or increased nutrient losses.

Specific nutrient deficiencies are not uncommonly encountered in patients with Crohn's disease involving the colon, although nutrient deficiencies are less common in patients with disease limited to the colon. Vitamin B_{12} deficiency is common in patients with disease affecting the terminal ileum, where this vitamin is absorbed. Patients may manifest deficiency in the face of a normal serum B_{12} concentration, and measurement of the serum methylmalonic acid (MMA) concentration is generally more sensitive. It is elevated in B_{12} deficiency. Because of steatorrhea resulting from fat maldigestion (caused by decreased bile salt re-absorption in the terminal ileum with subsequently decreased micelle formation), fat soluble vitamin (A, D, E, K) may occur. Serum concentrations of vitamin A, D (25-OH), E, and the prothrombin time are generally accurate reflections of nutrient status. Water soluble vitamin deficiency is less common, but folate and vitamin C deficiency can be seen.

Calcium supplements (1000 to 1500 mg/day) should be provided for patients taking corticosteroids because of decreased calcium absorption and increased calcium losses. Electrolyte depletion (K, Mg) may occur because of significant diarrheal losses. Oral Mg supplements are often cathartic, and periodic intramuscular or intravenous replacement may be required. Iron deficiency is common due to chronic blood loss. Low serum ferritin concentration is observed in iron deficiency. However, ferritin is an acute phase reactant, and as such, it may be *elevated*, and not reflect the iron deficient state. Zinc deficiency occurs frequently in patients with chronic diarrhea or small intestinal fistulas. A combination of low serum zinc and low urinary zinc concentrations generally reflects zinc deficiency. Oral zinc sulfate (200 mg/day) should be provided to correct deficiency.

Nutritional support may be provided as either primary therapy or as supportive therapy. For supportive therapy, the goal is to correct and to prevent nutrient deficiencies. Dietary restriction is only necessary in patients with short bowel syndrome or in patients with intestinal obstruction, in whom a low residual diet should be used, or, in the presence of high grade obstruction, the patient should be made NPO and consideration given to the provision of nutrients parenterally depending on the likely outcome. In ulcerative colitis, there may be some benefit from the use of diets high in soluble fiber because these fibers are metabolized by colonic bacteria to short chain fatty acids such as butyrate, which may have some effect on colonic healing. The incidence of lactose intolerance is no greater in patients with irritable bowel disorder (IBD) than in the general population except in the rare situations where duodenal or jejunal Crohn's disease is present. Because lactose-containing foods are an excellent source of Ca, lactose should be restricted only in patients with documented lactase deficiency.

For patients who require surgical resection of small intestine, preoperative TPN may improve outcome, although this should not be provided routinely and should not delay surgery in otherwise, well-nourished or only mildly depleted patients. In general, the indications for TPN include bowel obstruction, ileus or toxic megacolon, gastrointestinal hemorrhage, severe diarrhea and malabsorption, enterocutaneous or entero-enteric fistulas, and as supportive care in patients with moderately-severe or severe malnutrition that do not tolerate sufficient enteral nutrition.

The use of nutritional support for primary therapy may take several forms:

- Dietary supplementation with fish oils or oily fish may have some value in the treatment and/or prevention of relapse in patients with either Crohn's disease or ulcerative colitis, although the results of studies are inconclusive.
- "Bowel rest" and the provision of TPN may be useful in selected patients with severe Crohn's disease involving the small bowel, although not in patients

with disease primarily involving the colon, and in patients with enterocutaneous and entero-enteric fistulas, although the long-term remission rate and fistual closure rate is not particularly encouraging.

- Defined-formula enteral diets, provided for 3 to 6 weeks, may have benefit in the treatment of patients with Crohn's disease involving the small bowel, with remission rates approaching that of corticosteroids. However, data also suggest that less expensive and generally more palatable polymeric formula are associated with similar remission rates. There may also be some value in the provision of diets low in long-chain triglycerides and polyunsaturated fats.

REFERENCES

1. Leonard CD, Luke RG, Siegel RR. Parenteral essential amino acids in acute renal failure. *Urology.* 1975;6:154-7.
2. Feinstein EI, Blumenkrantz. Clinical and metabolic responses to parenteral nutrition in acute renal failure; a controlled double-blind study. *Medicine.* 1981;60:124-37.
3. Frankenfield DC, Badellino MM, Reynolds HN. Amino acids loss and plasma concentration during continuous hemodiafiltration. *JPEN.* 1993;17:551-61.
4. Goldstein S, Askanazi J, Thomashaw B, et al. Metabolic demand, ventilation and muscle function during repletion of malnourished COPD and surgical patients. *Anesthesiology.* 1985;63:A276.
5. Arora NS, Rochester DF. Respiratory muscle strength and maximal voluntary ventilation in undernourished patients. *Am Rev Resp Dis.* 1982;126:5-8.
6. Doekel RC, Zwillich CW, Scoggin CH, et al. Clinical semi-starvation: depression of hypoxic ventilatory response. *N Engl J Med.* 1979;295:358-361.
7. Weissman C, Askanazi J, Rosenbaum S, et al. Amino acids and respiration. *Ann Intern. Med.* 1983;98:41-4.
8. Newman JH, Neff TA, Ziporin P. Acute respiratory failure associated with hypophosphatemia. *N Engl J Med.* 1977; 296:1101-3.
9. Aubier M, Murciano D, Lecocguic Y. Effect of hypophosphatemia on diaphragmatic contractility in patients with acute respiratory failure. *N Engl J Med.* 1985;313:420-4.
10. Grevelyn TR, Brophy N, Siegert C, et al. Hypophosphatemia-associated respiratory muscle weakness in a general inpatient population. *Int J Surg.* 1982;67:371-2.
11. Venus B, Patel CB, Mathru M, Sandoval ED. Pulmonary effects of lipid infusion in patients with acute respiratory failure. *Crit Care Med.* 1984;12 293-294.

SUGGESTED READING

Afonso JJ, Rombeau JL. Nutritional care for patients with Crohn's disease. *Hepato-gastroenterol.* 1990;37:32-41.

Belluzzi A, Brignola C, Campieri M, et al. Effect of enteric coated fish oil preparations on relapses in Crohn's disease. *NEJM.* 1996;334:1557-1560.

Bousvaros A, Zurakowski D, Duggan C, et al. Vitamins A and E serum levels in children and young adults with inflammatory bowel disease: effect of disease activity. *J Ped Gastro Nutr.* 1999;26:129-134.

Buchman AL. Short bowel syndrome. In Bayless T, Diehl AM. *Advanced Therapy of Gastroenterology and Liver Disease.* 5th ed. Philadelphia: Lippincott; 2003.

Buchman AL, Scolopio J. Nutritional support in inflammatory bowel disease. In Lichtenstein GR. *The Clinician's Guide to Inflammatory Bowel Disease.* Thorofare, NJ: SLACK Incorporated; 2002:141-162.

Buchman AL, Scolopio J, Fryer J. Technical review of the treatment of short bowel syndrome and intestinal transplantation. *Gastroenterology.* 2003;124:1111-1134.

Dickinson RJ, Ashton MG, Axon AT, et al. Controlled trial of intravenous hyperalimentation and bowel rest as an adjunct to routine therapy of acute colitis. *Gastroenterology.* 1980; 79:1199-1204.

Fernandez-Banares F, Hinojosa J, Sanchz-Lombrana JL, et al. Randomized clinical trial of Plantago ovata seeds (dietary fiber) as compared with mesalamine in maintaining remission in ulcerative colitis. *Am J Gastroenterol.* 1999; 94:427-433.

Gonzalex-Huix F, de Leon R, Fernandez-Banares F, et al. Polymeric enteral diets as primary treatment of active Crohn's disease: a prospective steroid controlled trial. *Gut.* 1993;34:778-82.

Greenberg GR. Nutritional management of inflammatory bowel disease. *Semin Gastrointest Dis.* 1993;4:69-86.

Greenberg GR, Fleming CR, Jeejeebhoy KN. Controlled trial of bowel rest and nutritional support in the management of Crohn's disease. *Gut.* 1988;29:1309-1315.

Jones VA. Comparison of total parenteral nutrition and elemental diet in induction of remission of Crohn's disease. *Dig Dis Sci.* 1987;32:100-7.

Lashner BA, Evans AA, Hanauer SB. Preoperative total parenteral nutrition for bowel resection in Crohn's disease. *Dig Dis Sci.* 1989;34:741-746.

Lochs SH, Meryn S, Marosi L, et al. Has total bowel rest have a beneficial effect in the treatment of Crohn's disease. *Clin Nutr.* 1983;2:61-64.

Lorenz-Meyer H, Nicolay C, Schulz B, et al. Omega 3 fatty acids and low carbohydrate diet for maintenance of remission in Crohn's disease: a randomized controlled multicenter trial. *Scand J Gastroenterol.* 1996;31:778-785.

McIntyre PB, Powell-Tuck J, Wood SR. Controlled trial of bowel rest in the treatment of severe acute colitis. *Gut.* 1986;27:481-5.

Mullen JL, Hargrove WC, Dudrick SJ, et al. Ten years experience with intravenous hyperalimentation and inflammatory bowel disease. *Ann Surg.* 1978;187:523-529.

O'Morain C, Segal AW, Levi AJ, et al. Elemental diet as primary treatment of acute Crohn's disease: a controlled trial. *BMJ.* 1984;288:1859-62.

Ostro MJ, Greenberg GR, Jeejeebhoy KN. Total parenteral nutrition and complete bowel rest in the management of Crohn's disease. *JPEN.* 1985;9:280-287.

Reilly J, Ryan JA, Stole W, et al. Hyperalimentation in inflammatory bowel disease. *Am J Surg.* 1976;131:192-200.

Rigaud D., Cosnes J, Le Quintree Y, et al. Controlled trial comparing two types of enteral nutrition in treatment of active Crohn's disease: elemental versus polymeric diet. *Gut.* 1991;32:1492-7.

Sitzmann JV, Converse RL, Bayless TM. Favorable response to parenteral nutrition and medical therapy in Crohn's colitis. *Gastroenterology.* 1990;99:1647-52.

Valberg LS, Flanagan PR, Kertesz A, et al. Zinc absorption in inflammatory bowel disease. *Dig Dis Sci.* 1986;31:724-731.

Appendix A
Tables

TABLE 1

Clinical Signs of Nutrient Deficiencies

Clinical Finding	Consider Deficiency	Comment
Hair		
Easily pluckable, sparse	Protein, biotin, zinc	Loss of scalp and body hair may also occur
Straight, dull	Protein	Hair will be fine and silky
Flag sign	Protein, copper	Reddening of normally black scalp; occurs in black-skinned children, possibly due to abnormal sebaceous gland activity
Coiled/corkscrew-like	Vitamin A, C	Due to follicular change; due to a keratinization disturbance and possibly abnormal sebaceous gland activity
Skin		
Xerosis	Essential fatty acid	Dryness of skin
Petechiae	Vitamin A, C	Pin-head sized hemorrhages
Pigmentation		
Desquamation	Niacin	Signs of pellagra distributed symmetrically in sun-exposed areas; also seen in hemochromatosis, an iron storage disease
Follicular hyperkeratosis	Vitamin A, possibly essentially fatty acid deficiency	Keratin plugs in follicles, sandpaper feel of skin
"Flaky-pain" dermatitis	Protein	
Subcutaneous fat loss, fine wrinkling	Protein-energy	Minimal fat reserves; low values for anthropometric indices
Poor tissue turgor	Water	
Edema	Protein, thiamine	Seen in protein-energy malnutrition with hypoalbuminemia and in wet beriberi due to thiamine deficiency

TABLE 1 CONTINUED

Clinical Signs of Nutrient Deficiencies

Clinical Finding	Consider Deficiency	Comment
Purpura (subcutaneous skin hemorrhage)	Vitamin C, K	
Perifollicular hemorrhage	Vitamin C	
Pallor	Folate, iron, B_{12}, copper	
Excessive hair growth	Protein-energy	Like fetal lanugo: noticeable in girl with anorexia nervosa; may be heat retaining mechanism
Tendency toward excessive bruising (ecchymoses)	Vitamin C, K	Due to increased fragility of capillary walls
Pressure Sores	Protein-energy	Common in pressure and bony points
Seborrheic dermatitis	Essential fatty acid, pyridoxine, Zinc	Also seen in acrodermatitis enteropathica due to a defect in zinc absorption
Poor wound healing	Protein-energy, zinc, and possibly essential fatty acids	Scrotal or vulvar in riboflavin deficiency; nasolabial in pyridoxine deficiency
Dermatitis	Biotin	
Dry scaling	Nonspecific	
Thickening of skin	Essential fatty acid	
Eyes		
Angular palpebritis	Riboflavin	Can lead to xerophthalmia in severe deficiency
Dull, dry conjunctiva (xerosis)	Vitamin A	Angular in riboflavin deficiency
Blepharitis	B vitamins	Wernicke's syndrome; prompt treatment necessary
Ophthalmoplegia	Thiamine	Softening of cornea
Keratomalacia	Vitamin A	Early evidence of deficiency
Bitot's spot	Vitamin A	
Corneal vascularization	Riboflavin	
Photophobia	Zinc	
Lips and Oral Structures		
Angular fissures, scars, or stomatitis	B-vitamins, iron, protein, riboflavin	Also seen with ill-fitting dentures Seen especially at corners of mouth
Cheilosis	B_6, niacin, riboflavin, protein	Also associated with altered sense of smell
Dysgeusia	Zinc	If not edentulous
Swollen, spongy, bleeding gums	Ascorbic acid	

TABLE 1 CONTINUED

Clinical Signs of Nutrient Deficiencies

Clinical Finding	Consider Deficiency	Comment
Tongue		
Magenta tongue	Riboflavin	Controversial; magenta color may also be due to poor general nutrition
Fissuring, raw glossitis	Niacin	Due to inadequate repair of epithelial tissues
Large size, swollen	Iodine, niacin	In niacin deficiency, the tongue can be deeply fissured
Fiery red tongue	Folate, B_{12}	Seen if anemia is not pronounced
Atrophic lingual papillae	Riboflavin, nacin	
Teeth		
Loss of dental fillings, dental caries	Vitamin C	Survy
Glands		
Parotid enlargement	Protein	Rare, seen in alcoholic patients
Thyroid enlargement	Iodine	Seen in areas where deficiency has not been corrected by table salt iodination
Hypogonadism, delayed puberty	Zinc	
Nails		
Spoon-shaped nails (koilonychia)	Iron	
Brittle, ridged, lined nails	Protein-energy	May be protein undernutrition
Heart		
Tachycardia, cardiomegaly, congestive heart failure	Thiamine (wet beriberi)	Wet beriberi associated with high output congestive heart failure
Decreased cardiac function	Phosphorous	
Cardiac arrhythmias	Magnesium, potassium	
Cardiomyopathy	Selenium, copper	Referred to as Keshan disease in the Orient. Occurrence in the United States with parenteral nutrition
Small heart, decreased output, bradycardia	Protein-energy	Prone to congestive heart failure during refeeding
Sudden failure, death	Ascorbic acid, thiamine	In ascorbic acid deficiency, death may be due to myocardium hemorrhage
Abdomen		
Hepatomegaly (fatty liver)	Protein, fatty acid	Also commonly seen in alcoholics
Wasting	Energy	Found in marasmus

TABLE 1 CONTINUED

Clinical Signs of Nutrient Deficiencies

Clinical Finding	Consider Deficiency	Comment
Bones and Joints		
Bone pain	Calcium, Vitamin D, C, phosphorous	Osteomalacia due to repeated pregnancies with poor Ca intake, little sunlight, steatorrhea
Muscles, Extremities		
Wasting	Protein-energy	Evidence in temporal area, dorsum of hand between thumb and index fingers, calf muscles
Edema	Protein	
Muscular twitching	Protein, thiamine	
Muscular pain	Selenium	
Muscle cramps	Sodium, potassium	
	Sodium, chloride	
Neurologic		
Ophthalmoplegia, footdrop	Thiamine	Wernicke's encephalopathy
Disorientation	Thiamine, sodium, water	Korsakoff's psychosis; confabulation occurs in thiamin-deficient alcoholics
Decreased position, vibratory sense, ataxia, optic neuritis	B_{12}	Subacute combined cord degeneration
Weakness, paresthesia of legs, Hyporeflexia	Thiamine, pyridoxine, Pantothenic acid, B_{12} Thiamine	Nutritional polyneuropathy, especially with alcoholism; "burning foot" syndrome with pantothenic acid deficiency
Mental disorders	Niacin, B_{12}	In untreated B_{12} deficiency, mental disorders may progress to severe psychosis
Convulsions	Pyridoxine, calcium, thiamine (infants), magnesium, phosphorous	
Depression, lethargy	Biotin, Vitamin C	
Nonketonic hyperosmolar syndrome	Fluid	
Hypersthesia	Sodium	Due to large glucose infusions
Peripheral neuropathy	Pyridoxine, Vitamin E	that result in an osmotic diuresis; occurs in TPN patients
Other		
Diarrhea	Niacin	
Delayed wound healing and tissue repair	Vitamin C, zinc, protein-energy, Zinc, fatty acid	
Anemia, pallor	Pyridoxine, B_{12}, iron, folate, Copper	

TABLE 1 CONTINUED

Clinical Signs of Nutrient Deficiencies

Clinical Finding	Consider Deficiency	Comment
Anorexia	B_{12}, sodium, thiamine, Vitamin C energy, biotin, magnesium,	
Fatigue, lassitude, apathy	Phosphorous, iron, potassium, sodium, Protein-energy, magnesium,	
Growth retardation	Zinc, Vitamin D, calcium	
Constipation	Thiamine	GI dysmotility
Glucose intolerance	Chromium	
Bleeding diathesis	Vitamin K	

TABLE 2

Average Weight Chart

Height		Men (kg)			Women (kg)		
Inches	Cm	Small Frame	Medium Frame	Large Frame	Small Frame	Medium Frame	Large Frame
58	147				46-50	46-55	54-60
59	150				47-51	50-60	55-61
60	152				47-52	51-57	55-62
61	155				48-54	52-59	57-63
62	157	58-61	60-64	62.7-68.2	49-55	54-60	58-65
63	160	59-61.8	60.4-65	63-69.5	50-56	55-61	60-69
64	163	60-62.7	61.3-65.9	64.5-71	52-58	56-63	61-69
65	165	60.9-63	62.2-67.2	65.4-72.7	53-59	58-64	62-70
66	168	61.8-64.5	63.2-68.6	66-74.5	55-60	59-65	63-72
67	170	62.7-65.9	64.5-70	67.7-76.3	56-62	60-67	65-74
68	172	63-67.3	65.9-71.3	69-78	56-62	62-68	66-80
69	173	64.5-68.6	67.3-72.7	70.4-80	57-63	69-70	68-77
70	178	65.4-70	68.6-74	71.8-81.8	58.6-64.5	64-71	69-79
71	180	66-71.3	70-75.4	73.2-83.6	60-65.9	66-72	70-80
72	183	67.7-72.7	71.3-77.2	74.5-85.4	61-67	67-74	72-81
73	185	69-74.3	73-79	76-87	63-69		
74	188	70.4-76.3	74.5-80.9	78-89.5			
75	191	71.8-78	75.9-83	80-92			
76	193	73.6-80	78-85	82-94			

Data compiled from Metropolitan Life Weight Chart, 1983.

TABLE 3

Arm Measurements: Percentiles of Upper Arm Circumference (mm) and Estimated Upper Arm Muscle Circumference (mm) for Whites of the United States Health Examination Survey 1 of 1971 to 1974

	Arm Circumference (mm)						Arm Muscle Circumference (mm)					
	5th	50th	95th	5th	50th	95th	5th	50th	95th	5th	50th	95th
Age (yr)	Males			Females			Males			Females		
1 to 1.9	142	159	183	138	156	177	110	127	147	105	124	143
2 to 2.9	141	162	185	142	160	184	111	130	150	111	126	147
3 to 3.9	150	167	190	143	167	189	117	137	153	113	132	152
4 to 4.9	149	171	192	149	169	191	123	141	159	115	136	157
5 to 5.9	153	175	204	153	175	211	128	147	169	125	142	165
6 to 6.9	155	179	228	156	176	211	131	151	177	130	145	171
7 to 7.9	162	187	230	164	183	231	137	160	190	129	151	176
8 to 8.9	162	190	245	168	195	261	140	162	178	138	160	194
9 to 9.9	175	200	257	178	211	260	151	170	202	147	167	198
10 to 10.9	181	210	274	174	209	265	156	180	221	148	170	197
11 to 11.9	186	223	280	185	224	303	159	183	230	150	181	223
12 to 12.9	193	232	303	194	237	294	167	195	241	162	191	220
13 to 13.9	194	247	301	202	243	338	172	211	245	169	198	240
14 to 14.9	220	253	322	214	252	322	189	223	264	174	201	247
15 to 15.9	222	264	320	208	254	322	199	237	252	175	202	244
16 to 16.9	244	278	343	218	258	334	213	249	296	170	202	249
17 to 17.9	246	285	347	220	264	350	224	258	312	175	205	257
18 to 18.9	245	297	379	222	258	325	226	264	324	174	202	245
19 to 24.9	262	308	372	221	265	345	238	273	321	179	207	249
25 to 34.9	271	319	375	233	277	368	243	279	326	183	212	264
35 to 44.9	278	326	374	241	290	378	247	286	327	186	218	272
45 to 54.9	267	322	376	242	299	384	239	281	326	187	220	274
55 to 64.9	258	317	369	243	303	385	236	278	320	187	225	280
65 to 74.9	248	307	355	240	299	373	223	268	306	185	225	279

Adapted from Frisancho AR. New norms of upper limb fat and muscle areas for assessment of nutritional status. *Am J Clin Nutr.* 1981;343-2540.

TABLE 4

Normal Values for Maximal Inspiratory and Expiratory Respiratory Pressure for Adults

	Maximal Inspiratory Pressure ($cm\ H_2O$)		Maximal Expiratory Pressure ($cm\ H_2O$)	
Age Range (yr)	**Male**	**Female**	**Male**	**Female**
20 to 54	124±22	87±16	233±42	152±27
55 to 59	103±16	77±13	218±37	145±20
60 to 64	103±16	73±13	209±37	140±20
65 to 69	103±16	70±13	197±37	135±20
70 to 74	103±16	65±13	185±37	128±20

Values represent mean ±SD.

Adapted from Black LF, Hyatt RE. Maximal respiratory pressures: Normal values and relationship to age and sex. *Am Rev Resp Dis.* 1969;696.

TABLE 5

Lower Limits of Acceptable Grip Strength Preoperatively*

Age	Female Grip Strength (kg)	Male Grip Strength (kg)
15	28	42
20	29	43
25	30	44
30	30	45
35	30	45
40	30	45
45	30	45
50	29	45
55	28	44
60	27	43
65	25	41
70	23	39
75	20	37
80	18	35
85	15	32
90	11	29
95	8	26

*85% Age-sex standard.

Reprinted with permission from the American Society for Parenteral and Enteral Nutrition (A.S.P.E.N.) from the following: Journal of Parenteral and Enteral Nutrition (KPEN); Table 5; 1989;13:30-33 "Hand Grip Dynamometry as a Predictor of Postoperative Complications." A.S.P.E.N. does not endorse the use of this material in any form other than it entirety.

TABLE 6

Triceps Skinfold Thickness

Triceps Skinfold Percentiles (mm_2)*

Age (yr)	Males								Females							
	n	5	10	25	50	75	90	95	n	5	10	25	50	75	90	95
1 to 1.9	228	6	7	8	10	12	14	16	204	6	7	8	10	12	14	16
2 to 2.9	223	6	7	8	10	12	14	15	208	6	8	9	10	12	15	16
3 to 3.9	220	6	7	8	10	11	14	15	208	7	8	9	11	12	14	15
4 to 4.9	230	6	6	8	9	11	12	14	208	7	8	8	10	12	14	16
5 to 5.9	214	6	6	8	9	11	14	15	219	6	7	8	10	12	15	18
6 to 6.9	117	5	6	7	8	10	13	16	118	6	6	8	10	12	14	16
7 to 7.9	122	5	6	7	9	12	15	17	126	6	7	9	11	13	16	18
8 to 8.9	117	5	6	7	8	10	13	16	118	6	8	9	12	15	18	24
9 to 9.9	121	6	6	7	10	13	17	18	125	8	8	10	13	16	20	22
10 to 10.9	146	6	6	8	10	14	18	21	152	7	8	10	12	17	23	27
11 to 11.9	122	6	6	8	11	16	20	24	117	7	8	10	13	18	24	28
12 to 12.9	153	6	6	8	11	14	22	28	129	8	9	11	14	18	23	27
13 to 13.9	134	5	5	7	10	14	22	26	151	8	8	12	15	21	26	30
14 to 14.9	131	4	5	7	9	14	21	24	141	9	10	13	16	21	26	28
15 to 15.9	128	4	5	6	8	11	18	24	117	8	10	12	17	21	25	32
16 to 16.9	131	4	5	6	8	12	16	22	142	10	12	15	18	22	26	31
17 to 17.9	133	5	5	6	8	12	16	19	114	10	12	13	19	24	30	37
18 to 18.9	91	4	5	6	9	13	20	24	109	10	12	15	18	22	26	30
19 to 24.9	531	4	5	7	10	15	20	22	1,060	10	11	14	18	24	30	34
25 to 34.9	971	5	6	8	12	16	20	24	1,987	10	12	16	21	27	34	37
35 to 44.9	806	5	6	8	12	16	20	23	1,614	12	14	18	23	29	35	38
45 to 54.9	898	6	6	8	12	15	20	25	1,047	12	16	20	25	30	36	40
55 to 64.9	734	5	6	8	11	14	19	22	809	12	16	20	25	31	36	38
65 to 74.9	1503	4	6	8	11	15	19	22	1,670	12	14	18	24	29	34	36

*Percentiles for Triceps Skinfold for Whites of the United States Health and Nutrition Examination Survey 1 of 1971 to 1974

The Lange caliper was used in these studies.

Adapted from Frisancho AR. New norms of upper limb fat and muscle areas for assessment of nutritional status. *Am J Clin Nutr.* 1981;34:2540.

Table 7

Percentiles for Triceps Skinfold Thickness in Elderly Men

Age Group (yr)	5%	50%	95%
50 to 59	7.5	12.6	21.8
60 to 69	7.7	12.7	23.1
70 to 79	7.3	12.4	20.6
80+	6.6	11.2	18.0

Adapted from Kuczmarski et al. Descriptive anthropometric reference for older Americans. *JADA*. 2000;100:59-66.

Table 8

Percentiles for Triceps Skinfold Thickness in Elderly Women

Age Group (yr)	5%	50%	95%
50 to 59	16.4	26.7	37.0
60 to 69	14.5	24.1	34.9
70 to 79	12.5	21.8	32.1
80+	9.3	18.1	28.9

Adapted from Kuczmarski et al. Descriptive anthropometric reference for older Americans. *JADA*. 2000;100:59-66.

TABLE 9

Non-Protein Calorie to Nitrogen Ratio of Standard Parenteral Nutrition Solutions

Dextrose Concentration (%)	Dextrose Calories Per Liter (kcal)	Non-Protein Calorie to Nitrogen Ratio For Amino Acid Concentration		
		2%	3.5%	4.25%
10	340	106	60	50
15	510	159	90	75
20	680	212	120	100
25	850	239	151	125
30	1020	318	181	150
35	1190	372	211*	175

*Not available as a standard solution.

Calories from parenteral fat emulsion must be included in calculating the final non-protein calorie to nitrogen ration: $\frac{\text{Dextrose Calories + Fat Calories}}{\text{Amino Acids (g)}} \times 6.25$ = ratio

TABLE 10

Electrolyte Requirements

	Adult (Pediatric)
Sodium*	80 to 130 mEq/day (3 to 4 mEq/kg/day) as chloride, acetate salt or phosphate
Potassium	70 to 150 mEq/day (2 to 3 mEq/kg/day) as chloride, acetate or phosphate salt
Calcium	1.8 to 2.7 g/day (60 to 90 mg/kg/day or 90-135 mEq/day) as gluconate salt
Magnesium*	0.25 to 0.35 mEq/kg/day (0.25 to 0.5 mEq/kg/day) as sulfate salt
Phosphorous	930 to 1390 mg/day or 30 to 45 mmol/day (47 to 70 mg/kg/day)

*Increased with large losses present in gastrointestinal disease

Mineral Conversion Factors

Ca	20 mg = 1mEq = 0.5 mmol
P	31 mg = 1 mmol
Na	23 mg = 1 mEq = 1 mmol
K	39 mg = 1 mEq = 1 mmol
Mg	12 mg = 1 mEq = 0.5 mmol
Cl	35 mg = 1 mEq = 1 mmol

Table 11

Food and Nutrition Board, National Academy for Sciences-National Research Council Recommended Daily Allowances/Adequate Intakes (1997, 1998, 2000, and 2001)

	Age	Median Weight (kg)	Fat Soluble Vitamins: Vit A (wg)	Vit D (wg)	Vit E (wg)	Vit K (wg)
Infants	<6 mo.	6	400	5	4	2.0
	6 to 12 mo.	9	500	5	5	2.5
Children	1 to 3 yr	13	300	5	6	30
	4 to 8	20	400	5	7	55
	9 to 13	28	600	5	11	60
Males	14 to 18	45	900	5	15	75
	15 to 18	66	900	5	15	120
	19 to 24	72	900	5	15	120
	25 to 50	79	900	5	15	120
	>51	77	900	10	15	120
Females	14 to 18	46	700	5	15	75
	15 to 18	55	700	5	15	90
	19 to 24	58	700	5	15	90
	25 to 50	63	700	5	15	90
	>51	65	700	10	15	90
Pregnant			770	5	15	90
Lactating			1300	5	19	90

Data adapted from the National Academy of Science.

Table 12

Food and Nutrition Board, National Academy for Sciences-National Research Council Recommended Daily Allowances/Adequate Intakes (1997, 1998, 2000, and 2001)

Water Soluble Vitamins

Age		Vit C (mg)	Thiamine (B1)(mg)	RiboFlavin (B_2)(mg)	Niacin (mg NE)*	Vit B_6 (mg)	Folate (wg)	Vit B_{12} (wg)	Biotin (wg)
Infants	<6 mo.	40	0.2	0.3	2	0.1	65	0.4	5
	6 to 12	50	0.3	0.4	4	0.3	80	0.5	6
Children	1 to 3	15	0.5	0.5	6	0.5	150	0.9	8
(yr)	4 to 8	25	0.6	0.6	8	0.6	200	1.2	12
	9 to 13	45	0.9	0.9	12	1.0	300	1.8	20
Males	14 to 18	75	1.2	1.3	14 to 16	1.3	400	2.4	25
(yr)	19 to 30	90	1.2	1.3	16	1.3	400	2.4	30
	35 to 50	90	1.2	1.3	16	1.3	400	2.4	30
	>51	90	1.2	1.3	16	1.7	400	2.4	30
Females	14 to 18	65	1.0	1.0	14	1.2	400	2.4	25
(yr)	19 to 30	75	1.1	1.1	14	1.3	400	2.4	30
	25 to 50	75	1.1	1.1	14	1.3	400	2.4	30
	>51	75	1.1	1.1	14	1.5	400	2.4	30
Pregnant		85	1.4	1.4	18	1.9	600	2.6	30
Lactating		120	1.4	1.6	17	2.0	500	2.8	35

*NE (niacin equivalent) = 1 mg niacin or 60 mg dietary tryptophan

Data adapted from the National Academy of Science.

TABLE 13

Food and Nutrition Board, National Academy for Sciences-National Research Council Recommended Daily Allowances (1997, 1998, 2000, and 2001)

Minerals

	Age	Ca (mg)	P* (mg)	Mg (mg)	Fe (mg)	Zn (mg)	I (mcg)	Se (mcg)	Cv (mcg)
Infants	<6	210	100	30	0.27	2	110	15	200
(mo)	7 to 12	270	275	75	11	3	130	20	200
Children	1 to 3	1300	460	80	7	3	90	20	340
(yr)	4 to 8	1300	500	130	10	5	90	30	440
	9 to 13	1300	1250	240	10	8	120	40	700
Males	14 to 18	1300	1250	410	12	11	150	55	890
(yr)	19 to 30	1200	700	400	10	11	150	55	900
	35 to 50	800	700	420	10	11	150	55	900
	>51	800	700	420	10	11	150	55	900
Females	14 to 18	1300	1250	360	15	8	150	55	890
	19 to 24	1200	700	310	15	8	150	55	900
	25 to 50	800	700	310 to 320	15	8	150	55	900
	>51	800	700	320	10	8	150	55	900
Pregnant		1000	700	310 to 320	30	12	220	60	1000
Lactating		1000	700	355	15	12	290	70	1300

Data adapted from the National Academy of Science.

TABLE 14

Approximate Electrolyte Concentration of Body Fluids (mEq/L)

Source	Adult Volume Per Day	Na	K	Cl	HCO_3
Gastric	2000* to	60	20	90	–
	2500^ ml	100	10	100	–
Pancreas	1000 ml	140	5	75	90
Bile	1500 ml	140	5	100	35
Small Bowel	3500 ml	140	15	100	25
Diarrhea	1000 to 4000 ml	60	30	45	45
Sweat	500 to 4000 ml	40 to 80	4	40 to 80	–

*pH less than 4

^pH greater than 4

TABLE 15

Electrolyte Abnormalities Associated With Parenteral Nutrition

Abnormality	Manifestations	Usual Causes
Hyponatremia	Weakness, confusion	Na depletion, SIADH, renal failure Seizures, lethargy, CHF
Hypernatremia	Weakness, confusion	Inadequate free lethargy, thirst H_2O intake
Hypokalemia	Weakness, cramps, cardiac ectopy	Inadequate intake, anabolic state
Hyperkalemia	Weakness, paresthesias, cardiac arrhythmias	Excess intake, renal failure, acidosis
Hypocalcemia	Tetany, seizures, osteomalacia	Inadequate intake, sepsis, renal failure
Hypercalcemia	Lethargy, confusion	Excess intake, polyuria
Hypophosphatemia	Weakness, confusion, CNS changes, decreased white blood cell (WBC) function	Inadequate intake, anabolic state
Hyperphosphatemia	Hypocalcemia, metastatic calcification	Excess intake, renal failure, acidosis
Hypomagnesemia	Hypocalcemia, renal potassium wasting	Inadequate intake, diuretics

TABLE 16

Signs and Symptoms of Trace Element Deficiencies

Trace Element	Signs and Symptoms
Zinc	Anorexia, growth depression, dermatitis, hypogeusia, alopecia, impaired wound healing, immune suppression, night blindness, hypogonadism
Copper	Anemia (microcytic) leukopenia, neutropenia, osteoporosis, hair and skin depigmentation, poor connective tissue, neuropathy
Manganese	Growth depression, bone deformities, B-cell degeneration, retarded growth of hair and nails, transient dermatitis in animals
Chromium	Impaired glucose tolerance(?), elevated serum lipids(?), peripheral neuropathy
Iron	Anemia (microcytic)
Molybdenum	Growth retardation, impaired methionine and uric acid metabolism in animals
Iodine	Thyroid disease (goiter, hypothyroidism, cretinism)
Selenium	Cardiomyopathy, pseudoalbinism, macrocytic anemia, myositis, growth retardation, (?) cancer, infection
Silicon	Impaired growth, skeletal deformities, and connective tissue formation in animals
Fluoride	Caries, osteoporosis (?)
Cobalt	Pernicious anemia
Nickel	Growth retardation, impaired lipid metabolism in animals
Vanadium	Growth depression, impaired reproduction and lipid metabolism in animals

TABLE 17

Classic Vitamin Deficiency States

Vitamins	Role	Deficiency State
Water-Soluble		
Thiamine (B_1)	Co-enzyme in oxidative decarboxylation reactions	Beriberi, cardiomyopathy, peripheral neuropathy, encephalopathy
Riboflavin (B_2)	Co-enzyme of flavoproteins (FMN and FAD) involved in electron transport, tissue oxidation	Angular stomatitis, glossitis, photophobia, tearing, seborrheic dermatitis, (nasolabial fold and scrotum)
Pantothenic acid	Precursor of co-enzyme A involved in synthesis and fatty acids and steroid hormones	"Burning feet" syndrome, fatigue, leg cramps, paresthesias
Niacin	Constituent of the co-enzymes	Pellagra (dementia, diarrhea, dermatitis)
Pyridoxine (B_6)	Co-enzyme involved in amino acid metabolism and DNA synthesis	Peripheral neuropathy, convulsions, glossitis, cheilosis, seborrheic dermatitis (eyes, nose, and mouth areas)
Biotin	Co-enzyme in carboxylation reactions	Dermatitis, alopecia, depression, muscle pain, paresthesias
Folic acid	Co-enzyme in amino acid metabolism and DNA synthesis	Anemia (macrocytic), stomatitis, Diarrhea
B_{12}	Co-enzyme in amino acid metabolism and DNA synthesis	Anemia (megaloblastic), Neuropathy and paresthesias, glossitis
C	Connective tissue formation Oxidation/reduction reactions	Scurvy (weakness, irritability, bleeding gums, arthralgias, loosening of teeth) delayed wound healing, petechiae
Fat-Soluble		
A	Retinal pigment formation Epithelial integrity	Xerophthalmia Keratomalacia, night blindness, delayed wound healing, sterility (males)
D	Calcium and phosphate homeostasis	Rickets, osteomalacia
E	Antioxidant	Neuropathy (paresis of gaze, gait disturbance, decreased proprioception)
K	Synthesis of prothrombin factors II, VII, IX, X	Hemorrhage

TABLE 18

Long-Term Central Venous Catheter and Care Chart

Catheter Type	Description	Placement/ Duration	Dressing Care/Hub Care	Heparin Flush	Clamps	Priming Volume	Special Considerations
Peripherally Inserted Central Catheter (PICC)	Silastic, silicone Elastomer CVC inserted peripherally via basilic or ante-cutibal vein into central circulation	By RN or MD at bedside. May stay in place up to 12 months or more	Steri-strips, gauze, and sterile transparent dressing q. week	150 units (100 U/ml) heparin per lumen q.d. when capped after meds, IVs	Use slide clamp on microbore extension set	0.6 ml	Change microbore extension set q.4-6 weeks using sterile gloves. Never power push solution through catheter, may cause rupture. May develop post-insertation phlebitis for 24-48h during first week after insertion. Treat with moist heat, rest, elevation of extremity. 90% resolve without catheter removal
Tunneled CVCs Single Lumen: Broviac Hickman Double Lumen: Hickman, Quinton, RAAF	Tunneled silastic CVC with Dacron cuff designed for long-term access (also known as right atrial catheter)	By MD in OR or surgical procedure May stay in place indefinitely	Gauze and tape q. 24-48h, sterile trans parent 1 to 3 x /wk 3x3 hub care 30 second 2% chlorhexidine	300 U (100 U/ml) heparin per lumen q.d. when capped or after meds, IVs	Use preattached clamps on CVC or smooth jawed green plastic clamps	0.3-1.8 ml	Appearance of Dacron cuff at exit site indicates dislodge

Adapted from UCLA Policies and Procedures.

Table 18 Continued

Long-Term Central Venous Catheter and Care Chart

Catheter Type	Description	Placement/ Duration	Dressing Care/Hub Care	Heparin Flush	Clamps	Priming Volume	Special Considerations
Groshong Single or double lumen Silastic, silicone	Same as tunneled CVC but with slit valve at end of line to prevent reflux of blood into catheter	By MD in OR or surgical procedure area. May stay in place indefinitely	Gauze and tape q 24 to 48 hr, sterile transparent 1.3 x/wk. 3x3 hub care. 30-second 2% chlorhexidine prep on ports	No heparin flush with 5 ml NS q.7 days when capped or after IV meds, fluids. Flush with 10 ml NS after blood draw. Flush with 20 ml NS prior to blood draw when TPN on	No clamps necessary because of slit valve	0.4 to 1.2 ml	Line has blue and white stripes on silastic, yellow and red adapters on ends. Does not require heparin flush. Cannot be used to draw blood
Subcutaneous Infusion Port	Small chamber with self-sealing silicone rubber septum attached to silastic catheter implanted subcutaneously, accessed through skin via Huber needle	By MD in OR or surgical procedure area. May stay in place indefinitely	Sterile transparent dressing q. 1 to 3x/wk. 3x3 hub care. 30-second 2% chlorhexidine prep on ports	500 units (U/ml) with 5 ml NS q month when not in use or after IV meds, fluids	When needle in heparin (100 u/ml) place, use slide clamp on microbore extension set	1.2 to 2.1 ml	Change Huber needle q.week. Confirm Huber needle placement prior to port use by aspiration of blood from port. Watch for bubbling leakage of fluid around port when flushing. Rotate site of needle to prevent fistula tract formation to port

Adapted from UCLA Policies and Procedures.

TABLE 18 CONTINUED

Long-Term Central Venous Catheter and Care Chart

Catheter Type	Description	Placement/ Duration	Dressing Care/Hub Care	Heparin Flush	Clamps	Priming Volume	Special Considerations
Short-Term: (peripherally inserted central catheter) Single Lumen Double Lumen Triple Lumen Quadruple Lumen (Ex: Arrowcath, Quadath)	Single or multi-lumen catheter made of stiff plastic such as polyurethane or vinylchloride, placed percutaneously for short-term access up to 3 weeks	By MD at bedside. May stay in place approximately 7-21 days	Gauze and tape q.24h, sterile transparent q. M.W.F.	300 units (100 U/ml) heparin per lumen q.d. when capped, after IV meds, fluids	Use slide clamp on CVC or extension set	0.3-0.6 ml	Recommended lumen usage: distal: CVP readings, blood products, general access, medical: TPN, IV fluids, proximal: general access, venous blood draws

Adapted from UCLA Policies and Procedures.

TABLE 19

Osmolalities of Parenteral Nutrients

Nutrient	Concentration	MOsm/kg
Dextrose	10%	505
	20%	1010
	30%	1515
	40%	2020
	50%	2525
	60%	3030
	70%	3535
Fat Emulsion	10%	276-300
	20%	258-350
Amino Acids	8.5%	810
	10%	1000
Sodium Chloride	4 mEq/mL	4.99
Sodium Acetate	2 mEq/mL	4.0
Potassium Chloride	2 mEq/mL	4.0
Potassium Acetate	2 mEq/mL	4.0
Calcium Chloride	1.36 mEq/mL	2.15
Calcium Gluconate	0.46 mEq/ml	0.295

TABLE 20

Calorie and Protein Chart for Selected Rates and Dextrose/Amino Acid Concentrations

Rate	Volume	Calories (kcal/day) Dextrose Concentrations		Protein (g/day) Amino Acid Concentrations		
(ml/hr)	(ml/day)	10%	25%	2%	3.5%	4.25%
42	1000	340	850	20.0	35.0	42.5
50	1200	408	1020	24.0	42.0	51.0
60	1440	490	1224	28.8	50.4	61.2
70	1680	571	1428	33.6	58.8	71.4
80	1920	653	1632	38.4	67.2	81.6
83	2000	680	1700	40.0	70.0	85.0
90	2160	734	1836	43.2	75.6	91.8
100	2400	816	2040	48.0	84.0	102.0
110	2640	898	2244	52.8	92.4	112.2
120	2880	979	2448	57.6	100.8	122.4
125	3000	1020	2550	60.0	105.0	127.5

TABLE 21

Energy Content of Parenteral Nutrients (kcal/ml)

Nutrient	% w/v (g/100 ml)	Kcal/ml
Dextrose monohydrate	7.5	0.26
(3.4 kcal/g)	10.0	0.34
	12.0	0.41
	12.5	0.425
	15.0	0.51
	17.5	0.595
	20.0	0.68
	25.0	0.85
	30.0	1.00
	40.0	1.38
Protein	1.0	0.04
(4 kcal/g)	2.2	0.09
	2.3	0.092
	2.5	0.10
	2.7	0.11
	3.0	0.12
	4.0	1.16
Fat	10.0	1.10
	20.0	2.00

Examples of parenteral nutrition solutions:

1. Dextrose 12%; amino acids 2.2%: 0.41 kcal/ml + 0.09 kcal/ml - 0.5 kcal/ml
2. Dextrose 20%; amino acids 3.0%: 0.58 kcal/ml + 0.12 kcal/ml - 0.8 kcal/ml

Table 22

Amino Acid Profiles of Standard Crystalline Amino Acid Solutions for Parenteral Use*

Amino acid	Travasol 10%	FreAmine III[†] 10%	Aminosyn[†a] 15%	Novamine[†] 15%
Essential amino acids (g/dL)				
Lysine	0.58	0.73	1.58	1.18
Troptophan	0.18	0.15	0.30	0.25
Phenylalanine	0.56	0.56	0.45	1.04
Methionine	0.40	0.53	0.26	0.75
Threonine	0.42	0.40	0.60	0.75
Leucine	0.73	0.91	1.50	1.04
Isoleucine	0.60	0.69	0.99	0.75
Valine	0.58	0.66	0.75	0.96
Non-essential amino acids (g/dL)				
	0.48	0.28	0.45	0.89
Histidine	–	–	–	0.57
Glutamate	0.68	1.12	1.08	0.89
Proline	–	–	–	0.33
Aspartate	0.50	0.59	0.80	0.59
Serine	1.15	0.95	1.53	1.47
Arginine	2.07	0.71	1.49	2.17
Alanine	1.03	1.40	0.75	1.04
Glycine	0.04	–	0.40	0.39
Tyrosine	–	<0.02	1.05	0.43
Cysteine			1.11	0.75
Glutamic acid				

*Values given for the most single concentrated solution available in each product line.

[†]Contains sodium bisulfite as a preservative. [a]Formula will become sulfite-free by 2004.

Aminosyn and Novamine data extrapolated to 10% solution equivalent.

TABLE 23

Amino Acid Profiles of Modified Crystalline Amino Acid Solutions for Specialized Parenteral Use*

	Increased Essential Amino Acids				Increased Branch-Chain Amino Acids				Neonatal Formula
Amino Acid	**Aminess® 5.2%**	**Aminosyn ®© RF 5.2%**	**Nephramine II ®© 5.4%**	**RenAmin® 6.5%**	**Aminosyn ®© HBC 7%**	**Branchamin® 4%**	**FreAmine®© HBC 6.9%**	**HepatAmine®© 8%**	**Trophamine®© 6%**
Essential amino acids (g/dL)									
Lysine	0.06	0.50	0.64	0.45	0.26	0	0.41	0.61	0.49
Tryptophan	0.18	0.16	0.20	0.16	0.08	0	0.09	0.07	0.12
Phenylalanine	0.82	0.73	0.88	0.49	0.23	–	0.32	0.10	0.29
Methionine	0.82	0.73	0.88	0.50	0.21	–	0.25	0.10	0.20
Threonine	0.38	0.33	0.40	0.38	0.27	–	0.20	0.45	0.25
Leucine	0.82	0.73	0.88	0.60	1.58	1.38	1.37	1.10	0.84
Isoleucine	0.52	0.46	0.56	0.50	0.79	1.38	0.76	0.90	0.49
Valine	0.60	0.53	0.64	0.82	0.79	1.24	0.88	0.84	0.47
Non-essential amino acids (g/dL)									
Histidine†	0.41	0.43	0.25	0.42	0.15	–	0.16	0.24	0.29
Glutamate	–	–	–	–	–	–	–	–	0
Proline	–	–	–	0.35	0.45	–	0.63	0.80	0.41
Aspartate	–	–	–	–	–	–	–	–	0
Serine	–	–	–	0.30	0.22	–	0.33	0.50	0.23
Arginine	–	0.60	–	0.63	0.51	–	0.58	–	0.73
Alanine	–	–	–	0.56	0.66	–	0.40	0.77	0.32
Glycine	–	–	–	0.30	0.66	–	0.33	0.90	0.22
Tyrosine	–	–	–	0.04	0.03	–	–	–	0.14
Cysteine	–	–	<0.02	–	–	–	<0.02	<0.02	<0.02
Taurine	–	–	–	–	–	–	–	–	0.015

*Value given for a single concentrated solution available in each product line.

† Histidine is considered essential for patients with renal failure.

Contains sodium bisulfite. Product mentions are not intended as endorsements.

TABLE 24

Average Daily Calories From Parenteral Fat Emulsion Dosing Regimens

Dosing	10% Fat		20% Fat			
Frequency	100 ml	500 ml	100 ml	200 ml	250 ml	500 ml
Q D	110	550	200	400	500	1000
Q O D	55	275	100	200	250	500
Q 3 D	37	183	67	114	167	333
1 day/wk	16	79	29	57	71	143
2 day/wk	31	157	57	114	143	286
3 day/wk	47	236	86	171	214	429
4 day/wk	63	314	114	229	286	571
5 day/wk	79	393	143	286	357	714
6 day/wk	94	471	171	343	429	857

TABLE 25

Comparison of Two Commercially Available Intravenous Lipid Emulsions

	Intralipid (Baxter, Deerfield, Ill)	Liposyn II (Ross, Columbus, Ohio)
Composition (g /100 ml,%)		
Egg yolk phospholipids	1.2	1.2
Glycerol	2.5	2.5
Soybean oil	10	10
Fatty acid content (%)		
Linoleic acid	54	54.5
Linolenic acid	8	8.3
Oleic acid	26	22.4
Palmitic acid	9	10.5
Stearic acid	2.5	4.2
Osmolality (mOsm)	280	300
Caloric density (kcal/mL)	1.1	1.1
Vitamin E and PUFA content		
Alpha-tocopherol (mg/dL)	<1	20.0
Gamma-tocopherol (mg/dL)	12.0	0
Vitamin E activity (mg/L)	1.4	20.0
(units/L)	2.1	29.8
PUFA (g/l)	62.0	77.0
Vitamin E: PUFA ratio	0.02	0.26

PUFA = polyunsaturated fatty acid.

TABLE 26

Composition of Parenteral Multiple Vitamin Formulations

Vitamin	Infuvite Adult Baxter, Deerfield, Ill	MVI-12 Pediatric AAI Pharma, Wilmington, NC	Infuvite Pediatric Baxter, Deerfield, Ill	MVI-12 AAI Pharma, Wilmington, NC
	10 ml in 2 vials	5 ml†	5 ml in 2 vials	5 ml
Vitamin A (RE)	3300	2300	2300	330
Vitamin D_3 (IU)	200	400	400	200
Vitamin E (IU)	10	7	7	10
Thiamine (mg)	6	1.2	1.2	3
Riboflavin (mg)	3.6	1.4	1.4	3.6
Niacinamide (mg)	40	17	17	40
Pyridoxine (mg)	6	1	1	4
Dexpanthenol (mg)	15	5	5	15
Vitamin C (mg)	100	80	80	100
Folic Acid (mcg)	600	140	140	400
Vitamin B_{12} (mcg)	5	1	1	5
Vitamin K (mcg)	150	200	0.2	0
Biotin (mcg)	60	20	20	60

†<1 kg: 30% of vial contents

1 to 3 kg: 65% of vial contents.

TABLE 27

Recommended Daily Intravenous Intake of Essential Trace Elements

	Stable Adult	Acute Adult Catabolic State*	Stable Adult With Intestinal Losses*
Zinc	2.5 to 4.0 mg	Additional 2.0 mg 400 g/kg	Add 12.2 mg/l small bowel fluid lost; 17.1 mg/l of stool or ileostomy output
Iodine	?	1.0 µg/kg/day	–
Copper	0.5 to 1.5 mcg	–20 µg/kg	–
Chromium†	10 to 15 mcg	–0.2 µg/kg	
Manganese†	0.15 to 0.8 mg	–1 µg/kg	–
Selenium‡	40 to 120 mcg	?	–
	Pre-Term Infant	**Term Infant**	**Children**
Zinc	400 mcg/kg/day	250 mcg/kg/day <3m 100 mcg/kg/day >3m	10 mcg/kg/d Max. 5000 mcg/day
Copper	20 mcg/kg/day	20 mcg/kg/day	20mcg/kg/day max. 300 mcg/day
Chromium	0.20 mcg/kg/day	0.20 mcg/kg/day	0.20 mcg/kg/day max. 5.0 mcg/day
Magnesium	1.0 mcg/kg/day	1.0 mcg/kg/day	2.0 mcg/kg/day max. 50 mcg/day
Selenium‡	2.0 mcg/kg/day	2.0 mcg/kg/day	2.0 mcg/kg/day max. 30 mcg/day

Frequent monitoring of blood concentrations in these patients is essential to provide proper dosage.

*American Medical Associaton, Department of Food & Nutrition. Guidelines for Essential Trace Element Preparations for Parenteral Use. Adapted from *JAMA*. 1979;241(19):2051-2054. *Amer J Clin Nutr.* 1988;48:1324-33.

† Deficiency state in humans not conclusively identified.

‡ Not described by the AMA

TABLE 28

Medications That Can Be Co-Infused With IV Fat Emulsions

Cefamandole sodium	Cefacolin sodium
Cefoxitin sodium	Clindamycin
Digoxin	Dopamine HCl
Erhtyromycin	Furosemide
Gentamycin	Heparin
Hydrocortisione sodium succinate	Isoproterenol HCl
Insulin (regular)	Lidocaine HCl
Methyldopate HCl (in NS)	Methylprednisolone sodium succinate
Metoclopramide	Norepinephrine HCl
Oxacillin sodium	Penicillin G sodium or potassium
Ticarcillin	Tobramycin

TABLE 29

Medications That May Be Piggybacked Into Amino Acid/Dextrose Solution

Albumin	Amikacin sulfate
Aminophylline	Azlocillin sodium
Aztreonam	Carbenicillin disodium
Cefamandole sodium	Cefoxitin
Cefoperazone sodium	Ceftriaxone sodium
Cefotaxime solution	Cefuroxime
Ceftazidime	Cephapirin sodium
Cephalothin sodium	Cimetidine
Cephradine	Clindamycin
Chloramphenicol	Cytarabine
Cyclophosphamide	Dobutamine
Digoxin	Doxycycline
Dopamine HCl	5-Fluorouracil
Erhtyromycin	Gentamicin
Furosemide	Hydrocortisone sodium succinate
Heparin	Imipenem
Hydromorphone HCl	Isoproterenol HCl
Insulin (regular)	Leucovorin calcium
Levarterenol bitartrate	Meperidine HCl
Methotrexate sodium	Methicillin sodium
Methylprednisolone sodium succinate	Methyldopate HCl in NS
Mezlocillin	Metoclopramide HCl
Morphine sulfate	Miconazole
Nafcillin sodium	Moxalactam sodium
Oxacillin sodium	Norepinephrine
Piperacillin	Penicillin G sodium or potassium
Tetracycline	Ranitidine
Tobramycin	Ticarcillin
Vancomycin	Urokinase

Table 30

Normal Nutritional Values in Children

Test	Normal Value	Exceptions
Protein		
Blood		
Serum albumin (g/dL)	≥3.5	≥2.5 to 3 for infant
Retinal binding protein (mg/dL)	3 to 6	2 to 3 children <9yr
Blood urea nitrogen (mg/dL)	7 to 22	
Thyroxin binding protein (mg/dL)	20 to 50	
Transferrin (mg/dL)	170 to 250	
Fibronectin (mg/dL)	30 to 40	
Urine		
Creatinine/height index	>0.9	
3-methyl histidine (uMol/kg)	3.2 ± 0.6 male 2.1 ± 0.4 female 4.2 ± 1.3 neonate	
3-methyl histidine (uMol/gm creatinine)	126 ± 32 male 92 ± 23 female 253 ± 78 neonate	
Hydroxyproline index	>2	
Vitamin A		
Plasma retinol (mg/dL)	≥30	
Plasma retinol binding protein (mg/dL)	2 to 3	
Vitamin D		
25-OH-D_3 (ng/ml)	>20	
Riboflavin		
Red cell gluthatione reductase simulation %	<20	
Vitamin B_6		
Red cell transaminases Plasma pyridoxal phosphate Xanthurenic acid excretion	Feasible and useful in all age groups but not readily available and not practical in children <9 years of age	
Folacin		
Serum folate (ng/ml)	>6	
Red blood cell folate (ng/ml)	>160	
Vitamin K		
Prothrombin time (seconds)	11 to 15	
Vitamin E		
Plasma alpha-tocopherol (mg/dL)	≥0.7	
Red blood cell hemolysis test (%)	≤10	
Vitamin C		
Plasma (mg/dL)	>0.2	
Leukocyte (mg/100 cells)	difficult to perform on children due to sample requirements	

TABLE 30 CONTINUED

Normal Nutritional Values in Children

Test	Normal Value	Exceptions
Thiamine		
Red blood cell transketolase stimulation (%)	<15	
Vitamin B_{12}		
Serum vitamin B12 (pg/ml)	≥200	
Absorption test	excretion of more than 7.5% of ingested labeled Vitamin B_{12}	
Phosphorous (mg/dL)	5 to 8	
Iron		
Hematocrit (%)	39	31 neonate 33 infant 36 child and menstruating females
Hemoglobin (g/dL)	14	11 neonate 12 infant 13 child and menstruating females
Serum ferratin (ng/ml)	10	
Serum iron (ug/dL)	>60	>30 neonate >40 infant >50 child <4 yr
Serum total iron bindiing capacity (ug/dL)	350 to 400	
Serum transferrin saturation (%)	>16	>12 infant 14 to 15 child <9yr
Serum transferrin (mg/dL)	170 to 250	<80 neonate
Erythrocyte protoporphyrin (ug/dL rbcs)	<70	<75 infant
Zinc		
Serum zinc (ug/dL)	60 to 120	
Erythrocyte zinc	erythrocytes contain approximately 10 times more zinc than plasma	

TABLE 31

Peripheral Parenteral Nutrition Solutions for Children

	Neonate/Infant	Child (1-10 yr)	Adolescent
Dextrose	12.5 gm	12.5 gm	12.5 gm
Amino Acids	2.2 gm	2.2 gm	2.2 gm
NaCl	(2.6 mEq) 2.6 mmol	(2.6 mEq) 2.6 mmol	(4 mEq) 4.0 mmol
KH_2PO_4-K_2HPO_4	(2.8 mmol K) 1.5 mmol P	(0.9 mmol K) 0.6 mmol P	(0.7 mEq K) 0.5 mmol P
Ca gluconate	(48 mg Ca) 1.2 mmol	(20 mg Ca) 0.5 mmol	(20 mg Ca) 0.5 mmol
$MgSO_4$	(6 mg Mg) 0.5 mEq	(9.6 mg Mg) 0.8 mEq	(12 mg Mg) 1.0 mEq
KCl	(0.2 mmol) 0.2 mmol	(0.8 mmol) 0.8 mEq	(2 mmol) 2.0 mEq
Total K	3.0 mEq or mmol	1.7 mEq or Mmol	2.7 mEq or mmol

(0.5 kcal/ml): components per dl (100 ml)

TABLE 32

Central Parenteral Nutrition Solutions for Children

	Neonate/Infant (0.5 kcal/ml)	Child (1-10 yr) (0.8 kcal/ml)	Adolescent (0.8 kcal/ml)
Dextrose	12.5 gm	20.0 gm	20.0 gm
Amino Acids	2.2 gm	3.0 gm	3.0 gm
NaCl	(2.6 mEq) 2.6 mmol	(3.8 mEq) 3.8 mmol	(6 mEq) 6.0 mmol
KH_2PO_4-K_2HPO_4	(1.8 mmol K) 1.2 mmol P	(1.5 mmol K) 1.0 mmol P	(0.7 mmol K) 0.5 mmol P
Ca gluconate	(48 mg Ca) 1.2 mEq	(36 mg Ca) 0.9 mmol	(20 mg Ca) 0.5 mmol
MgSO4	(6 mg Mg) 0.5 mmol	(9.6 mg Mg) 0.8 mEq	(12 mg Mg) 1.0 mEq
KCl	0.2 mEq	(1.3 mEq) 1,3 mEq	(3 mEq) 3.0 mmol
Total K	2.4 mEq or mmol	2.8 mEq or Mmol	3.7 mEq or mmol

TABLE 33

Recommended Admixtures for Children

Solution 1 (1.0 kcal/mL)	
Dextrose	14.0 gm
Amino acids (Novamine or Freamine III)	3.0 gm
NaCl (6.2 mEq)	6.2 mmol
$KH_2PO4\text{-}K_2HPO_4$ (1.2 mmol K)	0.8 mmol P
Ca gluconate (16 mg Ca = 0.8 mEq)	0.4 mmol
$MgSO_4$ (9.6 mg Mg = 0.8 mEq)	0.4 mmol
KCl (3 mEq)	3.0 mmol
Trace minerals	Appropriate for age
Vitamins	Appropriate for age
Fat emulsion (Intralipid)	4.0 gm
Heparin	1 U/ml
Solution 2 (1.5 kcal/mL)	
Dextrose	25.0 gm
Amino acids (Novamine or Freamine III)	4.0 gm
NaCl (9.4 mEq)	9.4 mmol
$KH_2PO_4\text{-}K_2HPO_4$ (1.2 mEq K)	1.2 mmol P
Ca gluconate (24 mg Ca)	0.6 mmol
$MgSO_4$ (14.4 mg Mg = 1.2 mEq)	0.6 mmol
KCl (3 mEq)	3.0 mmol
Trace minerals	Appropriate for age
Vitamins	Appropriate for age
Fat emulsion (Intralipid)	4.0 gm
Heparin	1 U/ml

Components per dl (100 ml)

TABLE 34

Home TPN Solutions for Children (0.8 kcal/ml)

Neonate/Infant		Child (1 to 10 yr)	
Dextrose	20.0 gm	Dextrose	20.0 gm
Amino Acids	2.5 gm	Amino Acids	3.0 gm
NaCl (2.6 mEq)	2.6 mEq	NaCl	3.8 (mEq)
KH_2PO_4-		KH_2PO_4-	
K_2HPO_4 (2.2 mmol K)	1.5 mmol	K_2HPO_4(1.5 mmol K)	1.0 mmol
Ca gluconate (48 mg Ca)	2.0 mEq	Ca gluconate (34 mg Ca)	1.7 mEq
$MgSO_4$ (9.6 mg Mg = 0.8 mEq	0.8 mEq	$MgSO_4$ (9.6 mg Mg =0.8 mEq)	0.8 mEq
KCl	0.2 mEq	KCl	1.3 mEq
Total K = 2.4 mEq or mmol		*Total K = 2.8 mEq or mmol*	
Trace Minerals	0.1 mL/kg/day	Trace Minerals	0.1 ml/kg/day
Vitamins (MVI-Pediatric)	1 vial/day	Vitamins (MVI-Pediatric)	1 vial/day
Heparin	1 U/ml	Heparin	1 U/l

Adolescent	
Dextrose	20.0 gm
Amino Acids	3.0 gm
NaCl	6.0 mEq
KH_2PO_4-	
K_2HPO_4 (0.7 mEq K)	0.5 mmol
Ca gluconate (20 mg Ca)	1.0 mEq
$MgSO_4$ (6 mg Mg = 0.5 mEq)	0.5 mEq
KCl	3.0 mEq
Total K = 3.7 mEq or mmol	
Trace Minerals (MTE 5)	4 ml/day
Vitamins (MVI 12)	1 vial/day
Heparin	1 U/ml
Vitamin K 10.0 mg added 1 x per week	

This home TPN solution is lower in Ca and P than the solution used in the hospital. The hospital solution cannot be used at home because during storage, calcium and phoshporous are likely to precipitate. Fat emulsions will be required if TPN is supplying greater than 50% of caloric needs and/or food intake is not providing 4% of calories as essential fatty acids.

Components per dl (100 ml)

TABLE 35

Composition of Milks

	Gram/100 ml			mg/100 ml			Source		Osmolality (mOsm/kg of H2O) and General Comments
	Pro	Fat	CHO	NA/K	Ca/P	Fe	CHO	Fat	
Human milk 21 kcal/30 ml	1.0	3.5	7.0	17/53	26/14	0.2	Lactose	Human milk fat	(280) Fe supplementation recommended. Whey:casein ratio 60:40
Whole cow's milk (18.8 kcal/30 ml)	3.3	3.3	4.6	51/146	120/95	TR	Lactose	Butterfat	(279) Not recommended for infants <1 yr of age. Whey:casein ratio 18:82
2% milk (15.1 kcal/30 ml)	3.4	2.0	4.9	51/157	124/97	TR	Lactose	Butterfat	(279) Used to moderately reduce calories and fat. Not recommended for infants <2yrs of age
Skim milk (10.8 kcal/30 ml)	3.5	0.2	5.0	53/169	126/103	TR	Lactose	Trace Butterfat	(279) Deficient in essential fatty acids. Not recommended for childran <2yrs of age
Evaporated whole milk (32 kcal/30 ml) undiluted	7.2	7.9	10.6	111/318	274/212	0.2	Lactose	Butterfat	Milk is diluted and sugar added to make a 20 calorie/oz formula
Goat's milk (21 kcal/30 ml)	3.6	4.2	4.5	51/208	136/112	TR	Lactose	Butterfat	(267) Casein more readily digested than casein in cow's milk

TABLE 36

Standard Milk-Based Formulas for Infants

	Gram/100 ml			mg/100 ml			Source		Osmolality (mOsm/kg of
	Pro	Fat	CHO	NA/K	Ca/P	Fe	CHO	Fat	H2O) and General Comments
Similac (Ross) (20 kcal/30 ml)	1.45	3.6	7.2	18/71	49/38	0.15 w/Fe 1.2	Lactose	Coconut oil, Soy oil	(300) Whey:casein ratio 18:82
Similac (24 kcal/30 ml)	2.2	4.3	8.5	28/107	73/57	0.18 w/Fe 1.5	Lactose	Coconut oil, Soy oil	(380) Whey:casein ration 18:82. Available for hospital use only
Similac conentrate mixed to 24 kcal/oz	2.6	4.3	8.5	28/107	73/84	1.4	Lactose	Coconut oil, Soy oil	Prepared from standard Similac; concentrate patient requires formula instruction prior to discharge
Similac 27 kcal/30 ml	2.5	4.8	9.5	31/121	82/64	1.4	Lactose	Coconut oil, Soy oil	(410) Whey:casein ratio 18:82
Enfamil (Mead Johnson) (20 kcal/30 ml)	1.5	3.8	6.9	18/72	52/35	0.1 w/Fe 1.3	Lactose	Palm Olein, Soy oil, Coconut oil, Sunflower oil	(300) Whey:casein ratio 60:40
SMA (Wyeth) (20 kcal/30 ml)	1.5	3.6	7.2	15/56	42/28	1.2	Lactose	Coconut oil, Safflower oil, Oleo, Soy oil	(300) Milk-based formula with low renal solute load. Whey:casein ratio 60:40
Gerber	1.5	3.6	7.3	16/65	43/24	1.0	Lactose Malto-dextrins	Palm oil, Soy oil, Coconut oil, Sunflower oil	(320) Whey:casein ratio 18:82
Good Start	1.6	3.4	7.3	16/65	43/24	1.0	Lactose Malto-dextrins Corn oil	Palm oil, Oleic, Safflower oil	(260) Hydrolyzed whey protein formula

Table 37

Soy-Based Formulas for Infants

	Gram/100 ml			mg/100 ml			Source		Osmolality (mOsm/kg of
	Pro	Fat	CHO	NA/K	Ca/P	Fe	CHO	Fat	H2O) and General Comments
Isomil (Ross) (20 kcal/30 ml)	1.8	3.7	6.8	30/73	71/51	1.2	Corn syrup solids, Sucrose	Soy oil, Coconut oil	(240) Soy protein isolate formula. Lactose-free formula
Isomil SF (Ross) 20 kcal/30 ml	1.8	3.7	6.8	30/73	71/51	1.2	Hydrolyzed corn starch Corn syrup solids	Soy oil Coconut oil	(180) Soy protein isolate formula. Lactose- and sucrose-free
Prosobee (Mead Johnson) (20 kcal/30 ml)	2.0	3.5	6.7	24/81	63/49	1.3	Corn syrup solids	Palm Olein Coconut oil Soy oil Sunflower oil	(200) Soy protein isolate formula. Lactose- and sucrose-free
Nursoy (Wyeth) (20 kcal/30 ml)	1.8	3.6	6.9	20/70	60/42	1.2	Sucrose	Oleo Coconut oil Safflower oil Soy oil	(244) Soy protein isolate formula. Lactose-free, no corn syrup solids
I-Soylac (Loma Linda) 20 kcal/30 ml	2.1	3.7	6.7	28/78	68/47	1.3	Sucrose Tapioca starch	Soy oil	206) Soy protein isolate formula. Corn-free. Lactose-free, Fe fortified
Soylac (Loma Linda) 20kcal/30 ml	2.1	3.7	6.7	29/78	63/37	1.3	Corn syrup solids	Soy Sucrose Soy oil	(273) Soy protein isolate formula. Lactose-free, Fe fortified

TABLE 38

Specialized Infant Formulas

	Gram/100 ml			mg/100 ml			Source		Osmolality (mOsm/kg of H2O) and General Comments
	Pro	Fat	CHO	NA/K	Ca/P	Fe	CHO	Fat	
Alimentum (Ross) (20 kcal/30 ml)	1.9	3.8	6.8	29/79	70/50	1.2	Sucrose, Modified tapioca starch	MCT oil, Safflower oil, Soy oil	(370) for malabsorption problems. Protein is casein hydrolysate with added amino acids. 50% fat from MCT oil
Nutramigen (Mead Johnson) (20 kcal/30 ml)	1.9	2.6	8.9	31/73	63/42	1.3	Corn syrup solids, Modified corn starch	Corn oil, Soy oil	(320) for malabsorption problems. Protein is casein hydrolysate with added amino acids
Pregestimil (Mead Johnson) (20 kcal/30 ml)	1.9	3.7	6.9	26/73	62/42	1.3	Corn syrup solids, Modified corn starch, Destrose	MCT oil, Corn oil, Soy oil, Safflower oil	(300) for malabsorption problems. Protein is casein hydrolysate with added amino aicds. 55% fat from MCT oil
Pregestimil (24 kcal/30 ml)	2.3	4.4	8.3	31/88	74/50	1.6	Same as Pregestamil 20 above	Same as Pregestamil 20 above	(360) for malabsorption problems. Patient needs formula instruction prior to discharge
Portagen Mead Johnson (20 kcal/30 ml)	2.3	3.2	7.7	37/83	63/47	1.3	Corn syrup solids Sucrose	MCT oil, Corn oil	(220) Medium chain triglyceride formula for LCT intolerance. Protein is sodium caseinate. 87% MCT oil
Lofenalac (Mead Johnson) (20 kcal/30 ml)	2.2	2.6	8.7	31/68	83/83	1.3	Corn syrup solids, Modified tapioca starch	Corn oil	(360) Low phenylalanine formula used in treatment of PKU. Protein is specially processed casein hydrolysate reduced in phenylalanine with other added amino acids
Phenyl-Free (Mead Johnson) 29 kcal/30 ml	3.3	1.1	10.7	66/223	55/37	1.9	Sucrose, Corn syrup solids, Modified tapioca starch	Corn oil, Coconut oil	Whey protein. Low calcium formula

TABLE 38 CONTINUED

Specialized Infant Formulas

	Gram/100 ml			mg/100 ml			Source		Osmolality (mOsm/kg of
	Pro	Fat	CHO	NA/K	Ca/P	Fe	CHO	Fat	H2O) and General Comments
Lacto-Free (Mead Johnson) (20 kcal/30 ml)	1.5	3.6	6.9	20/73	38/19	1.1	Corn syrup	Palm oil, Soy oil, Coconut oil, Sunflower oil	Protein provided as amino acids without phenylalanine
Similac PM 60/40 (Ross) (20 kcal/30 ml)	1.5	3.8	6.9	16/58	16/19	0.15	Lactose	Soy oil, Coconut oil	(200) for lactose intolerance, lactose-free, mild protein isolate. Whey:casein ratio 20:80
S-29 (Wyeth) (20 kcal/30 ml)	1.7	2.2	9.8	1.0/32	7/18	1.3	Lactose	Oleo, Coconut oil, Safflower oil, Soybean oil	(280) low renal solute load. Minerals comparable to human milk. Lactalbumin:casein and calcium:phosphorous ratios comparable to human milk. Low iron formula
Calcilo (XD) (Wyeth) (20 kcal/30 ml)	1.6	4.1	7.5	16/60		1.3	Lactose	Corn oil Coconut oil	(360) very low renal solute load. Whey protein

TABLE 39

Formulas Designed for Low Birth Weight Infants

	Gram/100 ml			mg/100 ml			Source		Osmolality (mOsm/kg of H2O) and General Comments
	Pro	Fat	CHO	NA/K	Ca/P	Fe	CHO	Fat	
Enfamil Premature, Iron-Fortified (Mead Johnson) (24 kcal/30 ml)	2.4	4.0	8.8	31/82	131/66	1.5* (low Fe 0.2)	Corn syrup solids, Lactose	Soy oil, MCT oil, Coconut oil	(310) for low birth weight infants. Available for hospital use only. Whey:casein ratio 60:40. 40% fat from MCT oil
Similac Special Care Iron-Fortified (Ross) (24 kcal/30 ml)	2.2	4.4	8.6	35/105	146/73	1.5 (low Fe 0.3)	Lactose Hydrolyzed corn starch	MCT oil, Soy oil, Coconut oil	(280) For low birth weight infants. Available for hospital use only. Whey:casein ratio 60:40. 50% fat from MCT oil. recommended vitamin D supplement 400 IU/d
Similac Special Care (Ross) (20 kcal/30 ml)	1.8	3.6	7.1	29/87	122/61	0.2	Lactose Hydrolyzed corn starch	MCT oil, Soy oil, Coconut oil	(235) Available for hospital use only
Similac Natural Care (Ross) (24 kcal/30 ml)	2.2	4.4	8.6	35/104	170/85	–	Lactose corn starch Hydrolyzed	MCT oil, Soy oil, Coconut oil	Designed to be mixed with human milk or to be fed alternately with human milk to low birth weight infants
Enfamil Human Milk Fortifier with EBM+ (Mead Johnson) @4 pk/100 ml)	1.7	3.5	9.7	27/68.6	116/59	0.2	Glucose polymers Lactose	–	(380) For low birth weight infants or infants with volume restriction on expressed breast milk. Available for hospital use only. Whey:casein ratio 60:40. Recommended mixture is 2 pk of fortifier/100 ml human milk for 24 hr, afterwards, increase to 4 pk/100 cc for full fortification. Does not contain iron

*also available as low iron formula

+ EBM = expressed breast milk

TABLE 40

Modular Formulas for Infants

	Gram/100 ml			mg/100 ml			Source		Osmolality (mOsm/kg of H2O) and General Comments
	Pro	Fat	CHO	NA/K	Ca/P	Fe	CHO	Fat	
RCF (Ross) (12.1 kcal/30 ml at normal dilution without CHO)	2.0	3.6	0	30/73	70/50	0.15	None	Soy oil, Coconut oil	(64 without added CHO). Used for those unable to tolerate the type or amount of carbohydrate in standard formulas. Should not be used without added carbohydrate
Product 80056 (Mead Johnson) (17 kcal/30 ml without added protein and/or amino acids)	0	2.6	8.3	19/71	63/35	1.3	Corn syrup Modified tapioca starch	Corn oil	Protein-free formula. For infants requiring specific mixtures of amino acids. Adequate protein or amino acids, sodium, and potassium must be added
Product 3232 A (Mead Johnson) (12.7 kcal/30 ml without added CHO)	1.9	2.8	2.8	29/73	63/42	1.3	Modified tapioca starch	MCT oil Corn oil	(250 without added CHO). Mono-and disaccharide-free powder for use with added carbohydrate. Used for disaccharidase deficiencies and for intractable diarrhea management.
ProViMin (Ross) (3.13 kcal/30 ml without added CHO or fat)	2.2	0	0	35/97	71/50	1.1	–	–	A protein/mineral modular formula for use in special feedings for infants intolerant of usual amounts or types of carbohydrate and/or fat present in conventional feedings. Appropriate amounts of CHO, fat essential vitamins, and fatty acids must be added.

TABLE 41

Infant Carbohydrate-Protein-Fat Modular Additives

Ingredient	Calories	Gram/ Tbsp	Source	Comments
Polycose Powder (Ross)	3.76/g	6	Glucose polymers	Carbohydrate, which provides lower osmolality and minimal sweetness
Polycose Liquid (Ross)	2/ml	15	Glucose polymers	Carbohydrate, which provides lower osmolality and minimal sweetness
Dextrose	3.8 g	10	Corn sugar	Anhydrous disaccharide used to increase calories
Fructose	4/g	10	Fruit sugar	Monosaccharide added to formula to increase calories for infants allergic to corn sugar or intolerant to other carbohydrates
Sucrose	4/g	12	Cane or beet sugar	Disaccharide added to formula to increase calories
Corn Syrup	2.9/g	3.8 ml	20	Corn syrup added to increase calories; contains corn syrup, sugar, vanilla and salt; 150 mg Na/100 g
Casac (Mead Johnson)	3.7 g	4.7	Calcium caseinate	Protein powder used to increase protein in formulas; 88% protein 1.6% calcium. 150 mg Na/100 g powder
Instant Nonfat Dry Milk Powder	3.6 g	4.3	Milk	Contains 0.35 g protein per gm powder; may be added to food or formula to increase protein and calorie content. 540 mg Na/100 gm powder. 1260 mg Ca/100 mg powder
Cornstarch	3.5 g	8	Corn	Slow release of carbohydrate; helpful in certain metabolic disorders to treat hypoglycemia
MCT oil (Mead Johnson)	7.7 ml	14	Lipid fraction of coconut oil	Mainly triglycerides of the C9 and C10 saturated fatty acids. Absorbed directly into portal system. Bile salts and lipase not necessary for digestion and absorption. Does not contain essential fatty acids. Non-emulsified so not recommended for long-term continuous drip feeds

TABLE 41 CONTINUED

Infant Carbohydrate-Protein-Fat Modular Additives

Ingredient	Calories	Gram/ Tbsp	Source	Comments
Corn oil	8.4 ml	14	Corn	Consists primarily of oleic and linoleic unsaturated fatty acids. Non-emulsified so not recommended for long-term continuous drip feeds
Safflower oil	8.4/ml	14	Safflower	Linoleic and oleic unsaturated fatty acids, non-emulsified so not recommended for long-term continuous drip feeds
Microlipid (Sherwood)	4.5 ml		Safflower oil	50% fat emulsion used as a supplementary source of calories. High in linoleic acid
Dry Infant Rice Cereal	4.23 g	3.5	Rice	May be added to formula to thicken and increase carbohydrate content; suggest 1 Tbsp/oz maximum. 1 Tbsp = 15 kcal, 0.3 mg protein
Enfamil Human Milk Fortifier (Mead Johnson)	14 in 4 packets		Corn syrup solids Whey proteins Sodium caseinate	For addition to human milk to increase calories, protein, Ca, P, Na, vitamins, other minerals and trace elements. Add 2 pkt/100 ml for 24 hr and next day increase to 4 pkg/100 ml for fortification. *See "Formulations Designed for Low Birth Weight Infants" on page 153.

TABLE 42

Average Protein and Calorie Content of Strained Baby Foods*

Product	Amount	Weight (g)	Measure (tbsp)	Calories (g)	Protein (g)	Fat (mg)	NA
Dry infant cereal	1 tbsp	3.6	1	15	0.3	0.1	1
Vegetables	4 oz jar	113	9	50	2.0	0.15	36
Fruits	4 oz jar	113	9	65	0.45 or 0.5	0.09	6.7
Meats	2.5 oz jar	71	5	80	9.0	4	42
Egg Yolk	2 14 oz jars	64	4.5	130	6.0	11	25

*Compiled from data supplied by Gerber Products Company, Fremont, Michigan, 1991.

TABLE 43

Drug-Nutrient Interactions

Drugs may interfere with nutrient absorption or metabolism by several mechanisms. For example, metronidazole may alter taste sensations. Penicillamine, clofibrate, amphetamines, cytotoxic agents, anticholinergics, and digoxin (toxic levels), may cause anorexia. Cyproheptadine, phenothiazines, benzodiazepines, tricyclic antidepressants, hypoglycemic agents, and corticosteroids may cause hyperphagia.

The following list offers a few examples where drugs may induce specific nutritional deficiencies or toxicities. The list is not meant to be all-inclusive.

A.	Cholestyramine Clofibrate Colestipol	Malabsorption of Vitamins A, D, K, and folate
B.	Colchicine Rapid potassium repletion	Vitamin B_{12} deficiency
C.	Methotrexate Sulfasalazine Trimethoprim Triamterene Oral contraceptives Phenytoin	Folate deficiency
	Ethanol	Also Vitamin B_1 and B_{12} deficiency
D.	Isoniazid Hydralazine Cycloserine Ethionamide Penicillamine L-dopa Oral contraceptives Aspirin Barbiturates Phenytoin	Pyridoxine (Vitamin B_6) deficiency. Isoniazid also associated with tryptophan and niacin deficiency
E.	Antibiotics	Vitamin K deficiency
F.	Antacids Laxatives Phenytoin Barbiturates	Vitamin D deficiency
G.	Salicylates Antacids H2 blockers	Iron deficiency
H.	Amphotericin Diuretics	Hypokalemia, Hypomagnesemia,
	Diuretics	Also hyponatremia
	Cisplatin	
	Cyclosporin	Also hypertriglyceridemia
I.	Steroids L-asparaginase	Hyperglycemia

TABLE 43 CONTINUED

Drug-Nutrient Interactions

J.	Pentamidine	Hypoglycemia
K.	Sucralfate	Hypophosphatemia
	Steroids	
	Antacids	
L.	Thiazide diuretics	Hypercalcemia
M.	Nanthiazide diuretics	Hypocalemia Probenecid

TABLE 44

Laboratory Values During Pregnancy

Laboratory Test	Normal Values Non-Pregnant	Pregnant	Findings in Deficiency During Pregnancy
Urinary acetone	Neg.	Faint pos. in am	Pos.
Serum total protein (g/100 ml)	6.5 to 8.5	6 to 8	>6
Serum alb (g/100 ml)	3.5 to 5	2.5 to 4.5	<3.5
BUN (mg/100 ml)	10 to 25	5 to 15	<5
Fasting glucose (mg/100 ml)	70 to 110	65 to 100	<65
2hr Postprandial glucose (mg/100 ml)	<100	<120 (plasma)	>120
Serum Ca (mEq/1)	4.6 to 5.5	4.2 to 5.2	<4.2 or normal
Serum P (mg/100 ml)	2.5 to 4.8	2.3 to 4.6	No change
Alk Phos (IU/I)	35 to 180	35 to 180	No change
Chol (mg/100 ml)	120 to 290	177 to 355	N/A
TG (mg/100 ml)	33 to 166	130 to 400	N/A
Serum folate (ng/ml)	5 to 21	4 to 14	<4
Vit B_{12} (pg/ml)	430 to 1025	Decreased	Decreased
Serum Fe (µg/ml)	>50	>60	<60
TIBC (µg/100/ml)	250 to 400	300 to 600	<450
% TIBC sat.	30	≥20	<16
Serum Zn (µg/100/ml)	65 to 115	55 to 80	±50
Urinary Zn (µg/day)	200 to 450	200 to 450	±150

Adapted from Aubrey RH, Roberts A and Ceunca VG. The assessment of maternal nutrition. *Clin Perinatal.* 1975;2:207-19.

TABLE 45

Sodium Content of Selected Medications

Drug	mg	MEq
Aminosalicylate Sodium, 1 g	108.7	4.7
Ampicillin Sodium, 1 g	66.7	2.9
Ampicillin Sodium, 1 g and Sulbactam, 0.5 g	115.0	5.0
Azlocillin Sodium, 1 g	50.0	2.17
Carbenicillin Disodium, 1 g	108.1 to 121.9	4.7 to 5.3†
Cefazolin Sodium, 1 g	46.0 to 48.3	2.0 to 2.1
Cefaperazone Sodium, 1 g	34.0	1.5
Cefotaxime Sodium, 1 g	50.5	2.2
Cefotetan Disodium, 1 g	80.0	3.5
Cefoxitin Sodium, 1 g	53.8	2.3
Ceftazidime, 1 g	53.8	2.3
Ceftizoxime sodium, 1 g	60.0	2.6
Ceftriaxone Sodium, 1 g	82.8	3.6
Cefuroxime Sodium, 1 g	54.2	2.4
Chloramphenicol Sodium Succinate, 1 g	51.8	2.3
Methicillin Sodium, 1 g	66.7	2.9
Mezlocillin Sodium, 1 g	42.6	1.85
Moxalactam Sodium, 1 g	88.0	3.8
Nafcillin Sodium, 1 g	66.7	2.9
Oxacillin Sodium, 1 g	64.4	2.8
Penicillin G Potassium, 1 million units	7.6	0.3
Penicillin G Sodium, 1 million units	46.0	2.0
Phenytoin Sodium, 1 g	88.0	3.8
Piperacillin Sodium, 1 g	42.6	1.85
Sodium Bicarbonate, 50 ml of 7.5%, 8.4%	1026, 1150	44.6,50.06
Sodium Iodide, 1 g	156.0	.8
Sodium Polystyrene Sulfonate, 1 g, oral	94.3‡	4.1‡
Thiopental Sodium, 1 g	86.8	3.8
Ticarcillin Disodium, 1 g	119.6‡	5.2†
Ticarcillin Disodium and Clavulanate Potassium, 1 g	109	4.75

*Product formulation and sodium content are subject to change by manufacturer.

†Sodium content per gram of free acid; actual vial content can be as high as 6.5 mEq/g.

‡Total sodium content; only approximately 33% is liberated in clinical use.

Adapted from Knoben JE, Anderson PO, eds. *Handbook of Clinical Drug Data*, 6th Ed. Drug Intelligence Publ, Hamilton, IL, 1988 and Parenteral and Enteral Nutrition Handbook (UCLA Medical Center).

TABLE 46

Adult Enteral Formulas

Product	Manufacturer	Form	(kcal/ml)	Protein Source	g Protein/l	Fat g/l	Fiber (g/ 1000 kcal)	Fiber Source	MCT:LCT Ratio	OSM
Standard										
Nutren 1.0	Nestle	Liquid	1.0	Caseinate	40	38	0	N/A	25:75	315-370
Nutren 1.5	Nestle	Liquid	1.5	Caseinate	40	45	0	N/A	50:50	510
Nutren 2.0	Nestle	Liquid	2.0	Caseinate	40	53	0	N/A	75:25	745
Isocal	Mead Johnson	Liquid	1.1	Caseinate, Soy	32	42	0	N/A	20:80	270
Isocal HN	Mead Johnson	Liquid	1.1	Caseinate, Soy	42	42	0	N/A	40:60	270
Comply	Mead Johnson	Liquid	1.5	Caseinate	40	41	0	N/A	20:80	460
Deliver 2.0	Mead Johnson	Liquid	2.0	Caseinate, Soy	38	51	0	N/A	30:70	640
IsoSource Std.	Novartis	Liquid	1.2	Soy	36	32	0	N/A	20:80	490
IsoSource HN	Novartis	Liquid	1.2	Soy	44	32	0	N/A	20:80	490
NovaSource 2.0	Novartis	Liquid	2.0	Caseinate	45	44	0	N/A	20:80	790
Ensure Plus HN	Ross	Liquid	1.5	Caseinate, Soy	42	33	0	N/A	N/A	525
Osmolite	Ross	Liquid	1.1	Caseinate, Soy	35	33	0	N/A	20:80	300
Osmolite HN	Ross	Liquid	1.1	Caseinate, Soy	42	33	0	N/A	20:80	300
Osmolite HN Plus	Ross	Liquid	1.2	Caseinate	46	33	0	N/A	20:80	360
TwoCal HN	Ross	Liquid	2.0	Caseinate	42	45	0	N/A	20:75	690

TABLE 46 CONTINUED

Adult Enteral Formulas

Product	Manufacturer	Form	(kcal/ml)	Protein Source	g Protein/l	Fat g/l	Fiber (g/1000 kcal)	Fiber Source	MCT:LCT Ratio	OSM
Probalance Diet	Nestle	Liquid	1.2	Caseinate	45	34	8	soy, gum arabic	20:80	350-400
Nutren 1.0 Fiber	Nestle	Liquid	2.0	Caseinate	40	38	14	soy	25:75	320-380
Ultracal	Mead Johnson	Liquid	1.1	Caseinate, Milk	42	37	14	cellulose, soy	N/A	360
Ultracal HN Plus	Mead Johnson	Liquid	1.2	Caseinate, Milk	45	33	8	cellulose, soy, acacia	30:70	370
FiberSource Std.	Novartis	Liquid	1.2	Caseinate	36	32	8	soy, guar gum	20:80	490
FiberSOurce HN	Novartis	Liquid	1.2	Caseinate	44	32	8	soy, guar gum	20:80	490
IsoSource 1.5	Novartis	Liquid	1.5	Caseinate	45	43	7	soy, guar gum	30:70	650
Jevity	Ross	Liquid	1.1	Caseinate	42	33	14	soy	20:80	300
Jevity Plus	Ross	Liquid	1.2	Caseinate	46	33	10	oats, soy, gum arabic, cellulose	20:80	450
Standard, Immune-Enhanced										
Immun-Aid	Hormel	Powder	1.0	Lactoalbumin, Amino acids	80	22	0	N/A	50:50	460
IntensiCal	Mead Johnson	Liquid	1.3	Casein, l-arginine	62	32	0	N/A	25:75	550
Impact	Novartis	Liquid	1.0	Casein	56	28	0	N/A	27:73	375
Impact with Fiber	Novartis	Liquid	1.0	Casein	56	28	0	soy, guar gum	27:73	375

TABLE 46 CONTINUED

Adult Enteral Formulas

Product	Manufacturer	Form	(kcal/ml)	Protein Source	g Protein/l	Fat g/l	Fiber (g/1000 kcal)	Fiber Source	MCT:LCT Ratio	OSM
Impact with Glutamine	Novartis	Liquid	1.3	Casein, whey protein hydrolysate	60	33	0	Soy, guar gum	27:73	630
Impact 1.5	Novartis	Liquid	1.5	Casein, l-arginine	56	46	0	N/A	55:45	550
Perative	Ross	Liquid	1.3	Casein, lactoalbumin hydrolysate, l-arginine	51	29	0	N/A	40:60	385
Replete	Nestle	Liquid	1.5	Hydrolyzed casein, l-arginine	62	34	0	N/A	25:75	300-350
Replete with Fiber	Nestle	Liquid	1.0	Casein	62	34	14	Soy	25:75	390
Protain XL	Mead Johnson	Liquid	1.0	Casein	57	30	9	Soy	20:80	340
TraumaCal	Mead Johnson	Liquid	1.0	Casein	55	45	0	N/A	30:70	560
Isosource VHN	Novartis	Liquid	1.0	Casein	62	29	10	Soy, guar gum	50:50	300
Promote	Ross	Liquid	1.0	Casein, Soy	62	26	0	N/A	20:80	340
Promote with Fiber	Ross	Liquid	1.0	Casein, Soy	62	28	14	oats, Soy	20:80	380

TABLE 46 CONTINUED

Adult Enteral Formulas

Product	Manufacturer	Form	(kcal/ml)	Protein Source	g Protein/l	Fat g/l	Fiber (g/1000 kcal)	Fiber Source	MCT:LCT Ratio	OSM
Peptide-Based or Free Amino Acids										
Crucial	Nestle	Liquid	1.5	Hydrolyzed Casein	63	45	0	N/A	50:50	490
Peptamen	Nestle	Liquid	1.0	Hydrolyzed Whey	40	39	0	N/A	70:30	270-380
Peptamen with FOS/Inulin	Nestle	Liquid	1.0	Hydrolyzed Whey	40	39	4	FOS, Inulin	70:30	290
Peptamen 1.5	Nestle	Liquid	1.5	Hydrolyzed Whey	45	37	0	N/A	70:30	550
Peptamen VHP	Nestle	Liquid	1.0	Hydrolyzed Whey	62	39	0	N/A	70:30	300-430
Reabilan	Nestle	Liquid	1.0	Hydrolyzed Casein, Whey	32	40	0	N/A	50:50	350
Reabilan HN	Nestle	Liquid	1.3	Hydrolyzed Casein, Whey	44	40	0	N/A	50:50	490
Criticare HN	Mead Johnson	Liquid	1.1	Hydrolyzed Casein, amino acids	36	5	0	N/A	N/A	650
Subdue	Mead Johnson	Liquid	1.0	Hydrolyzed Casein, whey	50	34	0	N/A	50:50	440-525
Subdue Plus	Mead Johnson	Liquid	1.5	Hydrolyzed Casein, whey	51	34	0	N/A	50:50	400
Sando-Source Peptide	Novartis	Liquid	1.0	Hydrolyzed Casein, amino acids	50	17	0	N/A	54:46	490
Vivonex TEN	Novartis	Powder	1.0	Amino acids	38	3	0	N/A	No MCT	630

TABLE 46 CONTINUED

Adult Enteral Formulas

Product	Manufacturer	Form	(kcal/ml)	Protein Source	g Protein/l	Fat g/l	Fiber (g/ 1000 kcal)	Fiber Source	MCT:LCT Ratio	OSM
Vivonex Plus	Novartis	Powder	1.0	Amino acids	45	7	0	N/A	No MCT	650
AlitraQ	Ross	Powder	1.0	Hydrolyzed Soy, whey, amino acids	52	16	0	N/A	53:47	575
Optimental	Ross	Liquid	1.0	Hydrolyzed Casein, Soy, arginine	51	28	5	FOS	N/A	540
Vital HN	Ross	Powder	1.0	Hydrolyzed Whey, Soy, Meat, amino acids	42	11	0	N/A	45:55	500
f-a-a-Free Amino Acid Diet	Nestle	Liquid	1.0	Amino acids	50	11	0	N/A	25:75	700
Glucose Intolerance										
Glytrol	Nestle	Liquid	1.0	Casein	45	48	15	Soy, pectin, gum arabic	20:80	380
Choice dm	Mead Johnson	Liquid	1.1	Milk Protein	42	48	12	Soy, acacia, cellulose	N/A	400
DiabetiSource	Novartis	Liquid	1.0	Casein, beef	50	49	4	vegetables, fruits	No MCT	360
ReSource Diabetic	Novartis	Liquid	1.1	Casein, Soy	59	44	11	guar gum, Soy	N/A	300-320
Glucerna	Ross	Liquid	1.0	Casein	42	54	14	Soy	No MCT	355
Hepatic Formulas										
Nutri-Hep	Nestle	Liquid	1.5	Amino acids, whey protein, (50% BCAA)			0	N/A	66:34	690
Hepatic Aid II	Hormel	Powder	1.2	Amino acids, (46% BCAA)			0	N/A	No MCT	560

TABLE 46 CONTINUED

Adult Enteral Formulas

Product	Manufacturer	Form	(kcal/ml)	Protein Source	g Protein/l	Fat g/l	Fiber (g/1000 kcal)	Fiber Source	MCT:LCT Ratio	OSM
Inflammatory Bowel Disease										
Modulen IBD	Nestle	Powder	1.0	Casein retain (processed to TGF-b2)			N/A	N/A	25:75	370
Pulmonary Formulas										
Nutrivent	Nestle	Liquid	1.5	Casein	45	63	0	N/A	40:60	330-450
NovaSource Pulmonary	Novartis	Liquid	1.5	Casein	50	45	8	Soy, guar gum	20:80	650
Respalor	Mead Johnson	Liquid	1.5	Casein	50	45	0	N/A	30:70	400
Oxepa	Ross	Liquid	1.5	Casein	42	62	0	N/A	25:75	493
Pulmocare	Ross	Liquid	1.5	Casein	42	62	0	N/A	20:80	475
Renal (Pre-Dialysis) Formulas										
Renalcal	Nestle	Liquid	2.0	Essential amino acids, select non-essential amino acids, whey protein	17	41	0	N/A	70:30	600
Amin-Aid	Hormel	Powder	2.0	Essential amino acids, histidine	10	23	0	N/A	No MCT	700
Suplena	Ross	Liquid	2.0	Casein	15	48	0	N/A	N/A	600
Renal (Dialysis) Formulas										
NutriRenal	Nestle	Liquid	2.0	Casein	35	52	0	N/A	50:50	650
Magnacal Renal	Mead Johnson	Liquid	2.0	Casein	38	50	0	N/A	20:80	570
NovaSource Renal	Novartis	Liquid	2.0	Casein, l-arginine	37	50	0	N/A	N/A	700-960
Nepro	Ross	Liquid	2.0	Casein, milk protein isolate	35	48	0	N/A	N/A	665
Re/Neph	Ross	Liquid	2.0	Casein, whey protein isolate	32	44	0	N/A	N/A	770

Appendix B Growth Charts

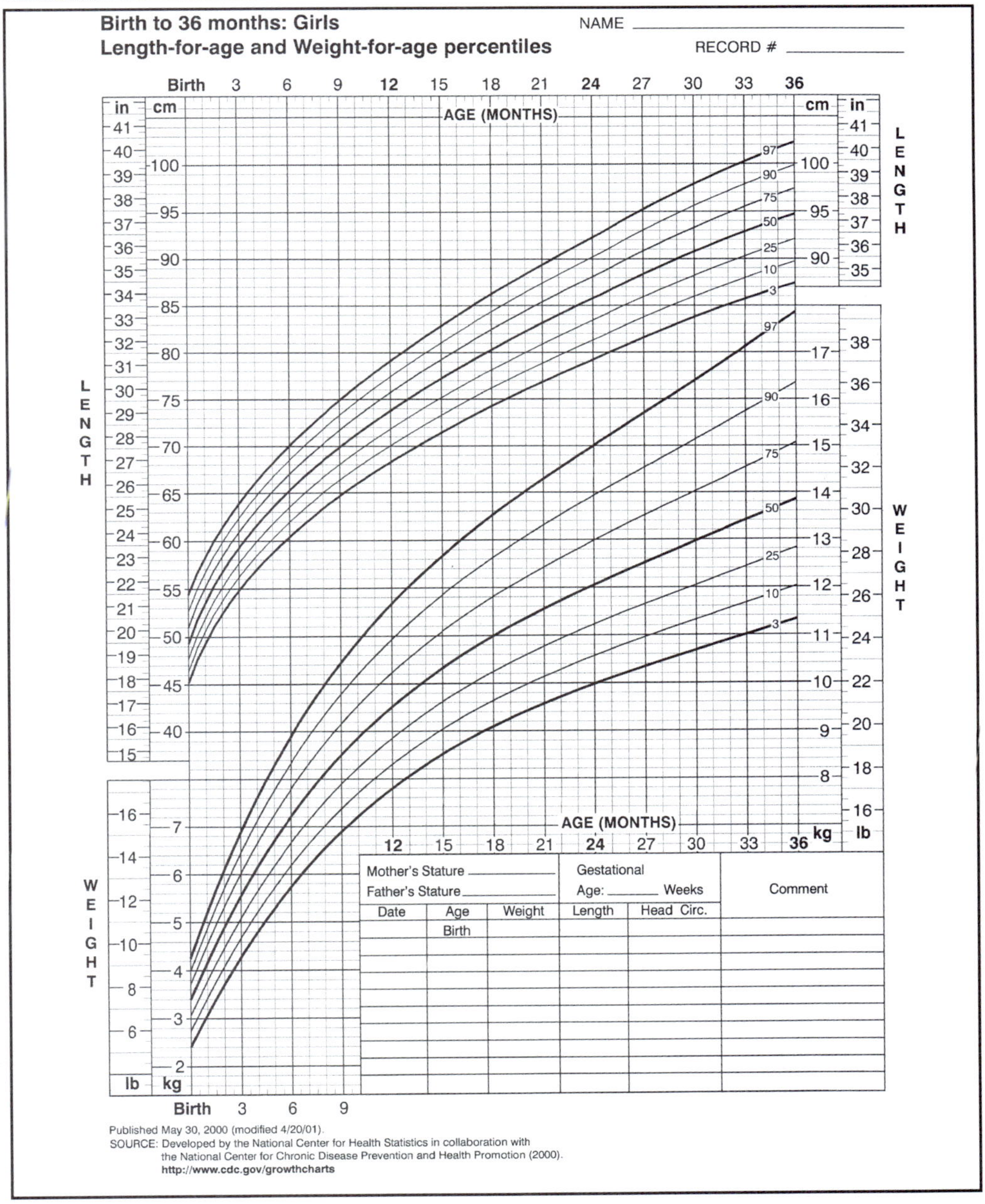

Figure 1. Girls: birth to 36 months length-for-age and weight-for age NCHS percentiles.

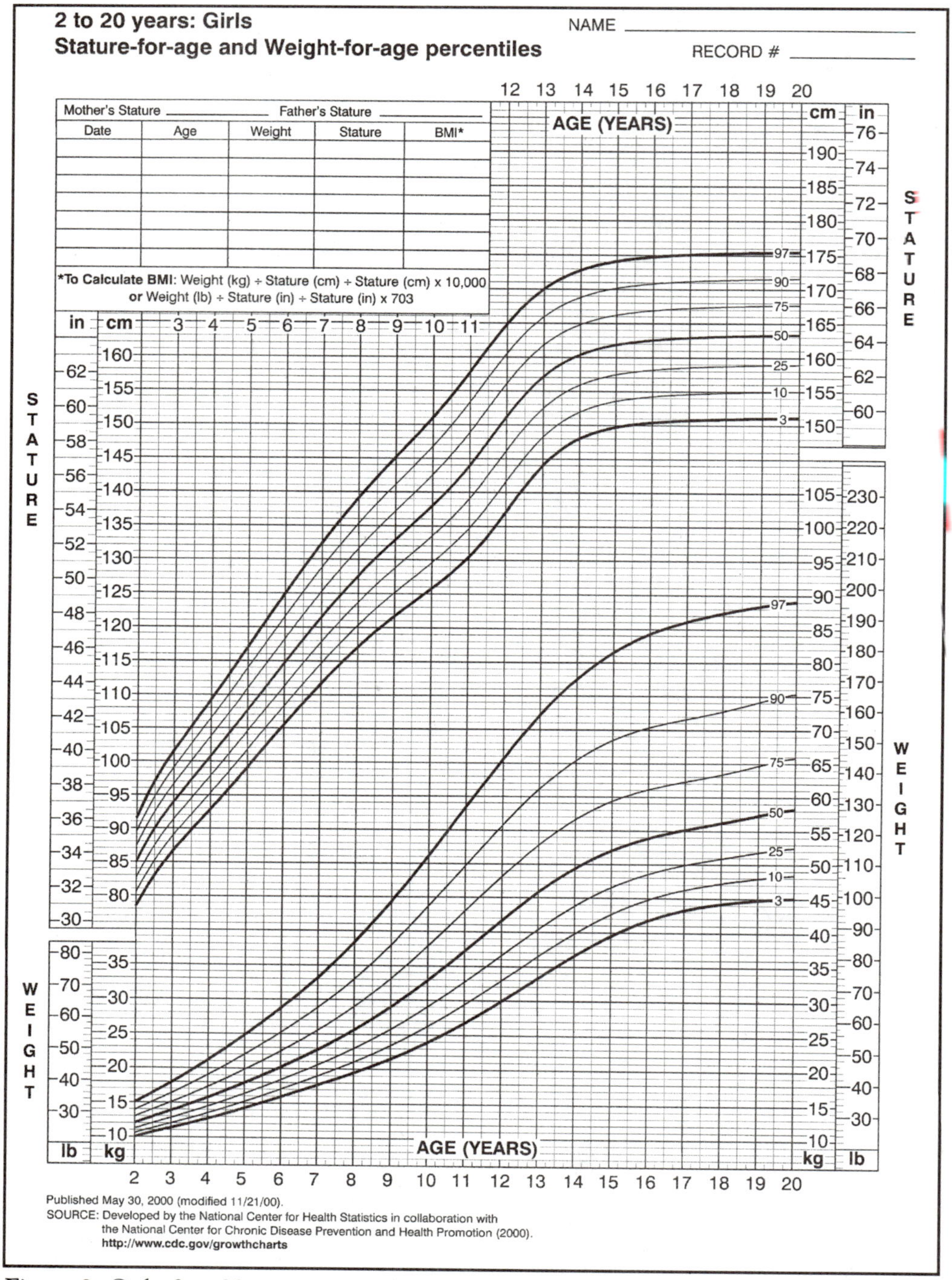

Figure 2. Girls: 2 to 20 years stature-for-age and weight-for age NCHS percentiles.

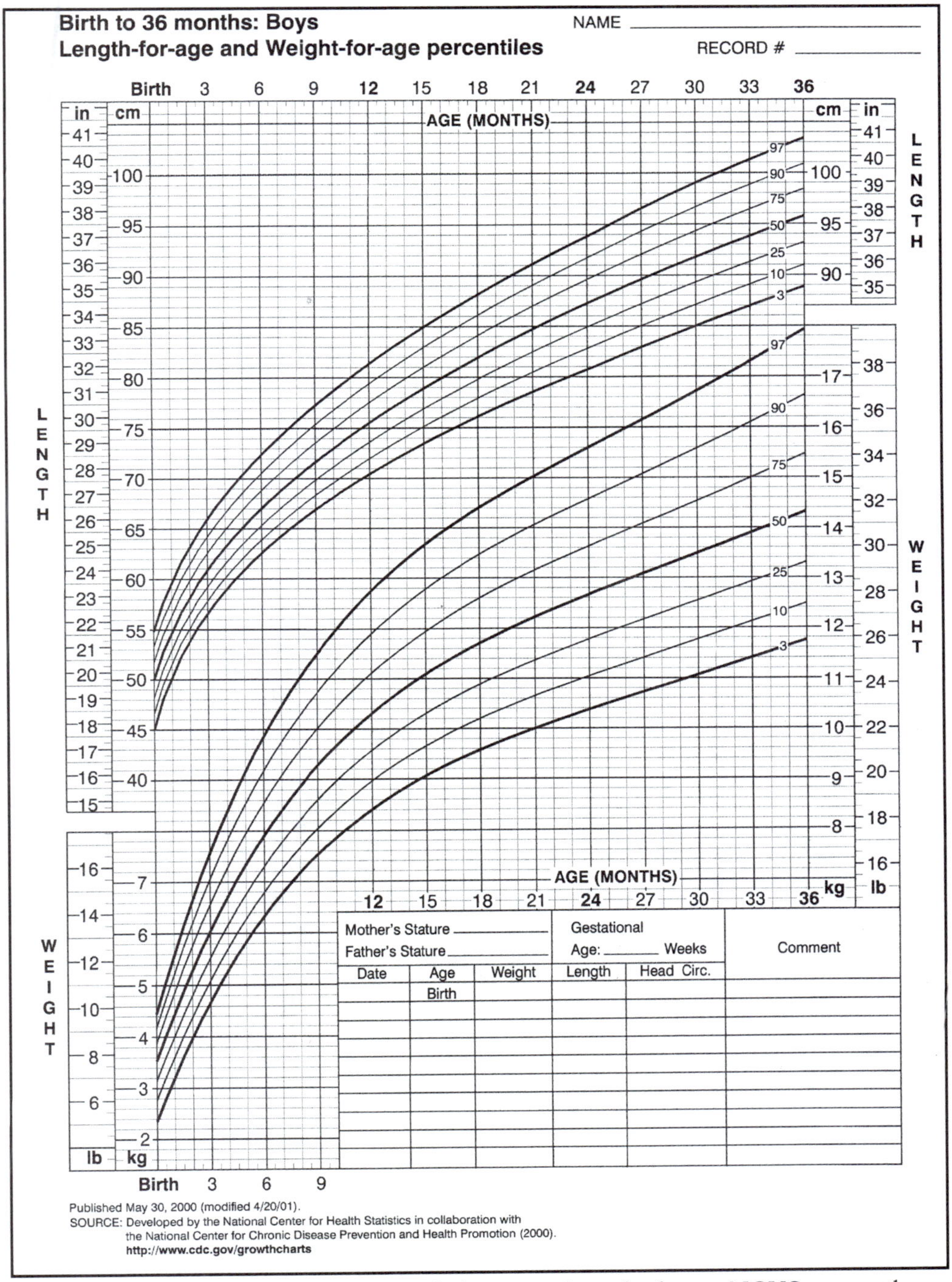

Figure 3. Boys: Birth to 36 months length-for-age and weight-for age NCHS percentiles.

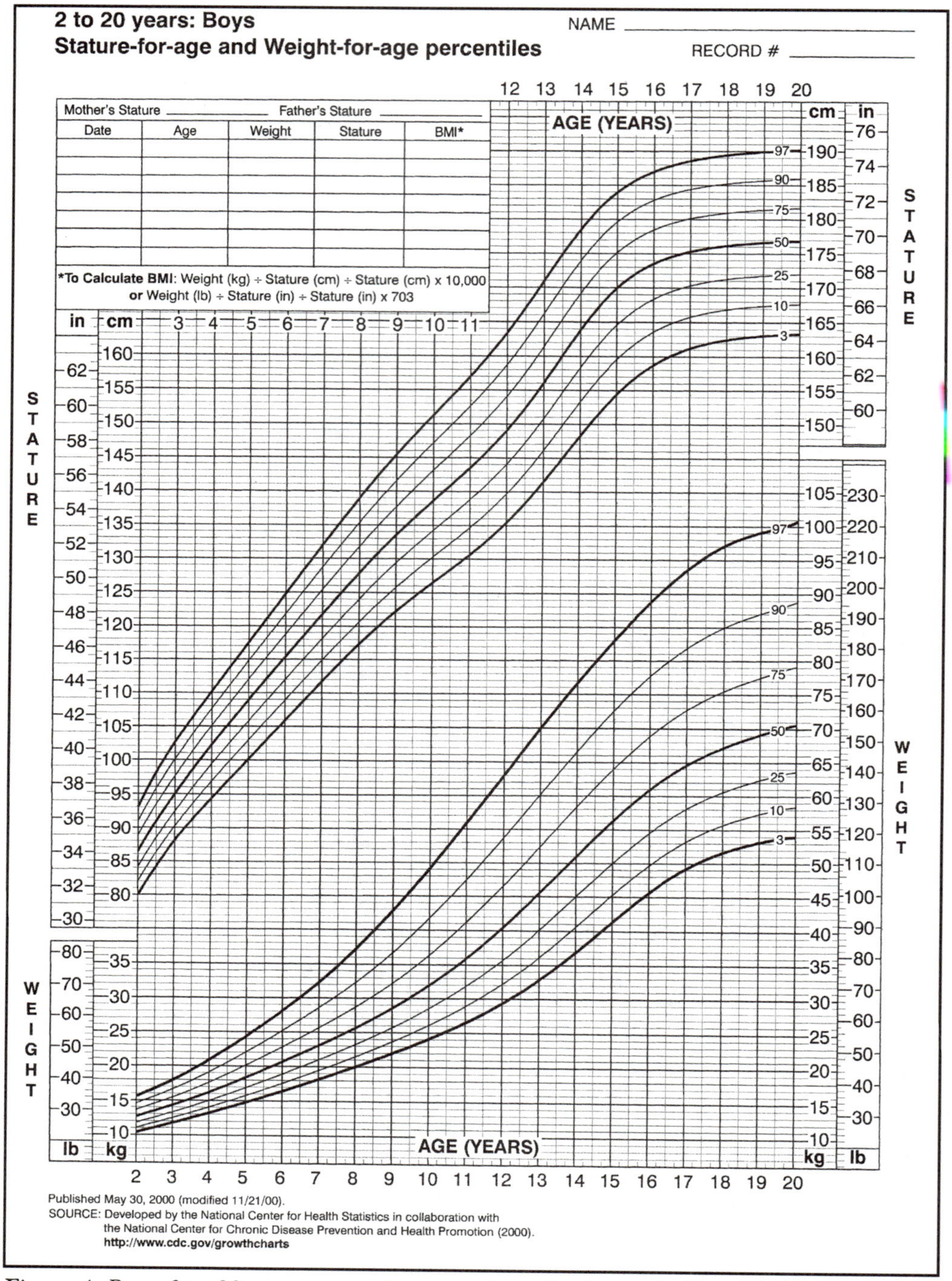

Figure 4. Boys: 2 to 20 years stature-for-age and weight-for age NCHS percentiles.

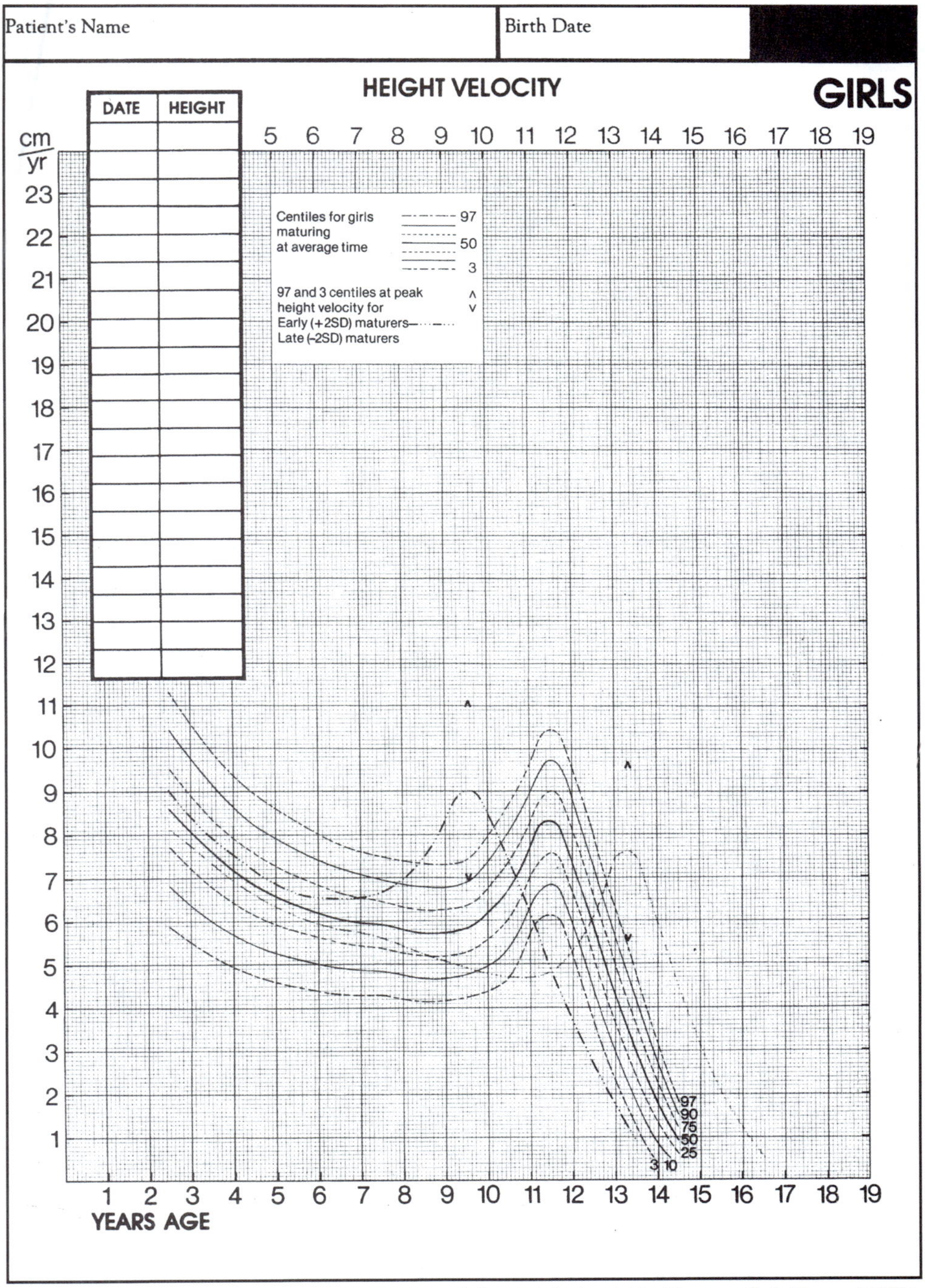

Figure 5. Height velocity, girls. (Reprinted from *J Peds,* 107, Tanner JM, Davis PSW. Clinical longitudinal standards for height and height velocity for North American children, 317-329, copyright 1985, with permission from Elsevier.)

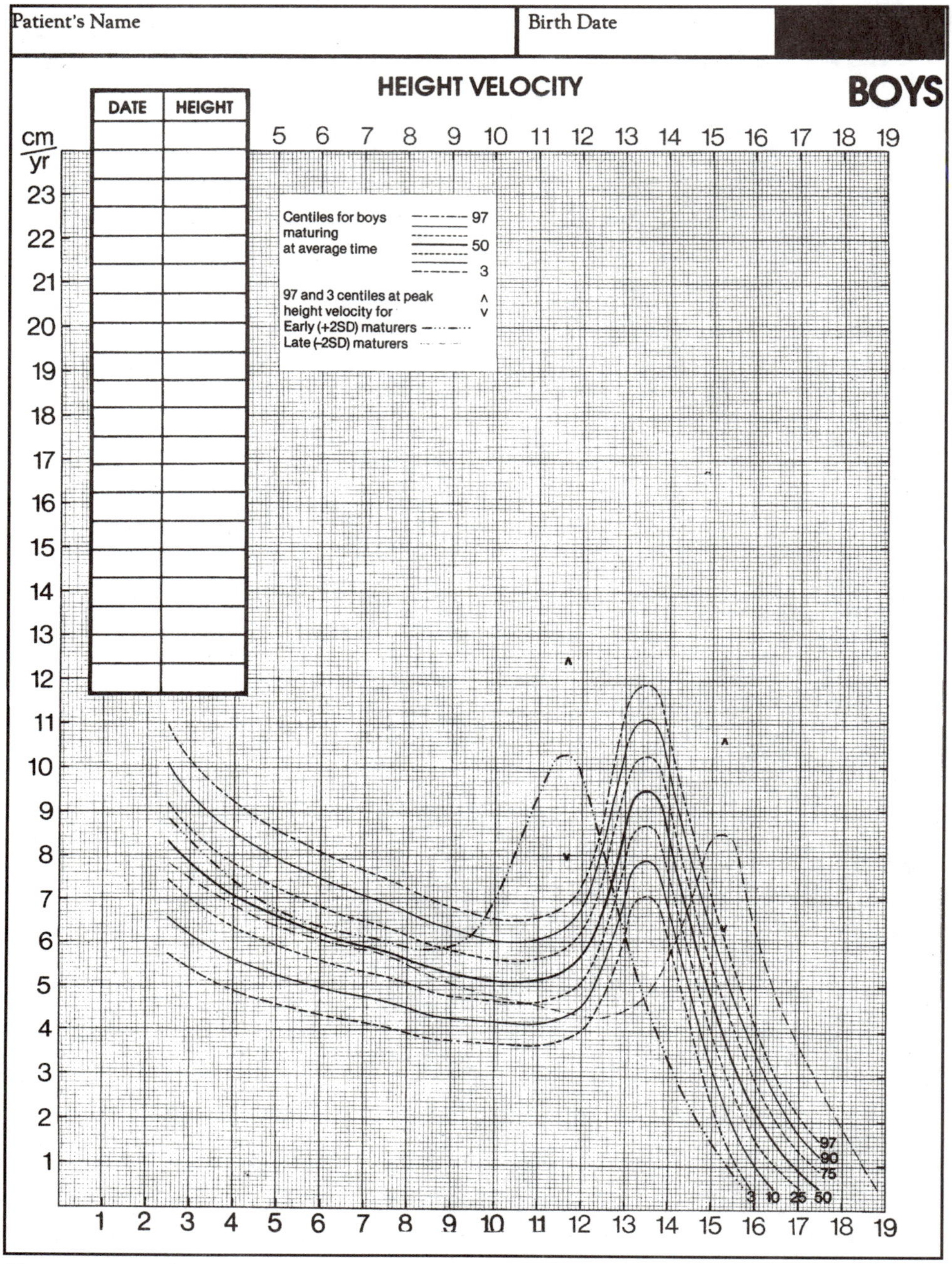

Figure 6. Height velocity, boys. (Reprinted from *J Peds*, 107, Tanner JM, Davis PSW. Clinical longitudinal standards for height and height velocity for North American children, 317-329, copyright 1985, with permission from Elsevier.)

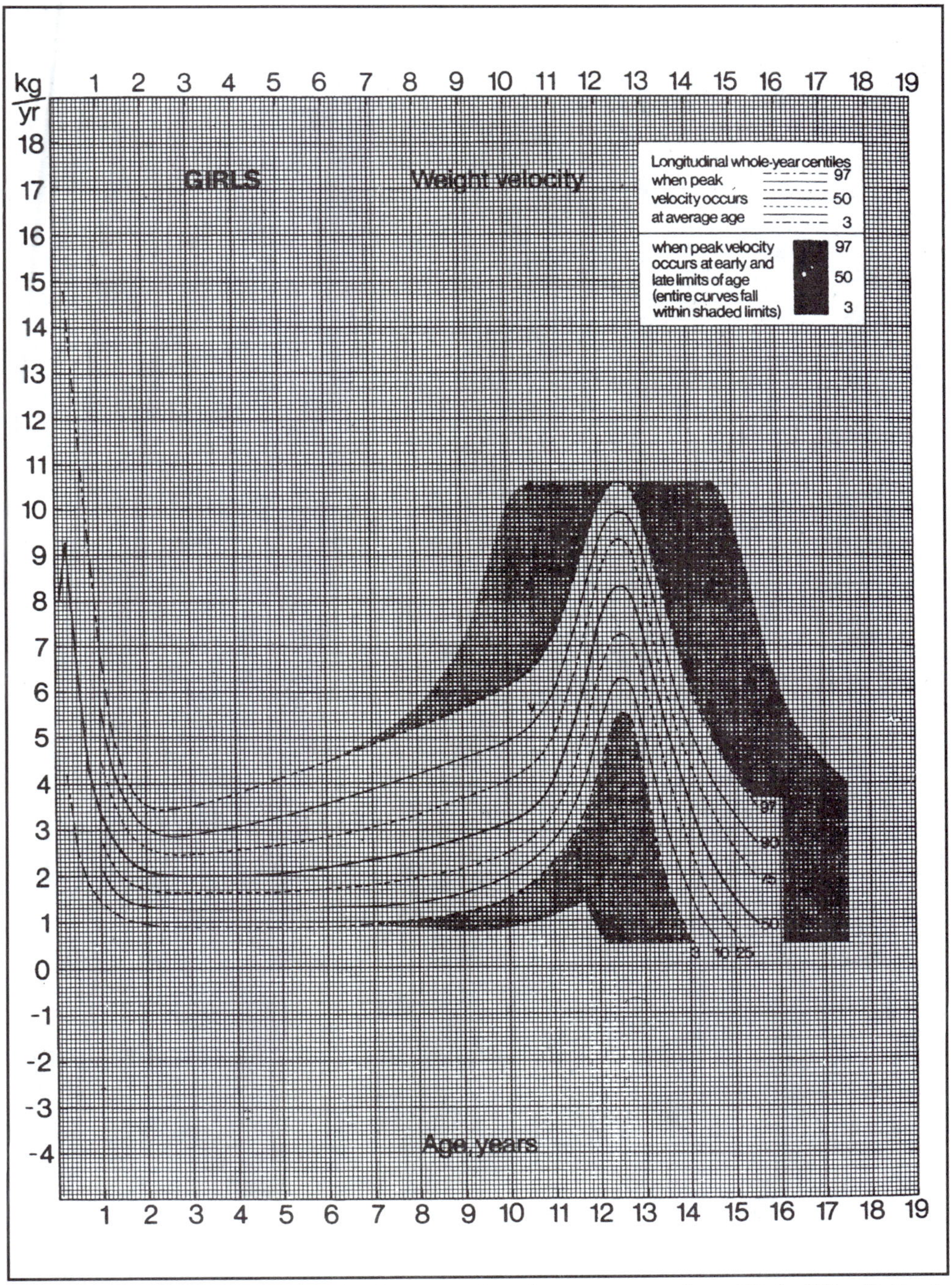

Figure 7. Weight velocity, girls. (Reprinted with permission from Klish WL, *Pediatric Gastrointestinal Disease-Pathophysiology, Diagnosis, Management*, Tanner JM, Whitehouse RH (eds), 1098-1099, copyright 1993, with permission from Elsevier).

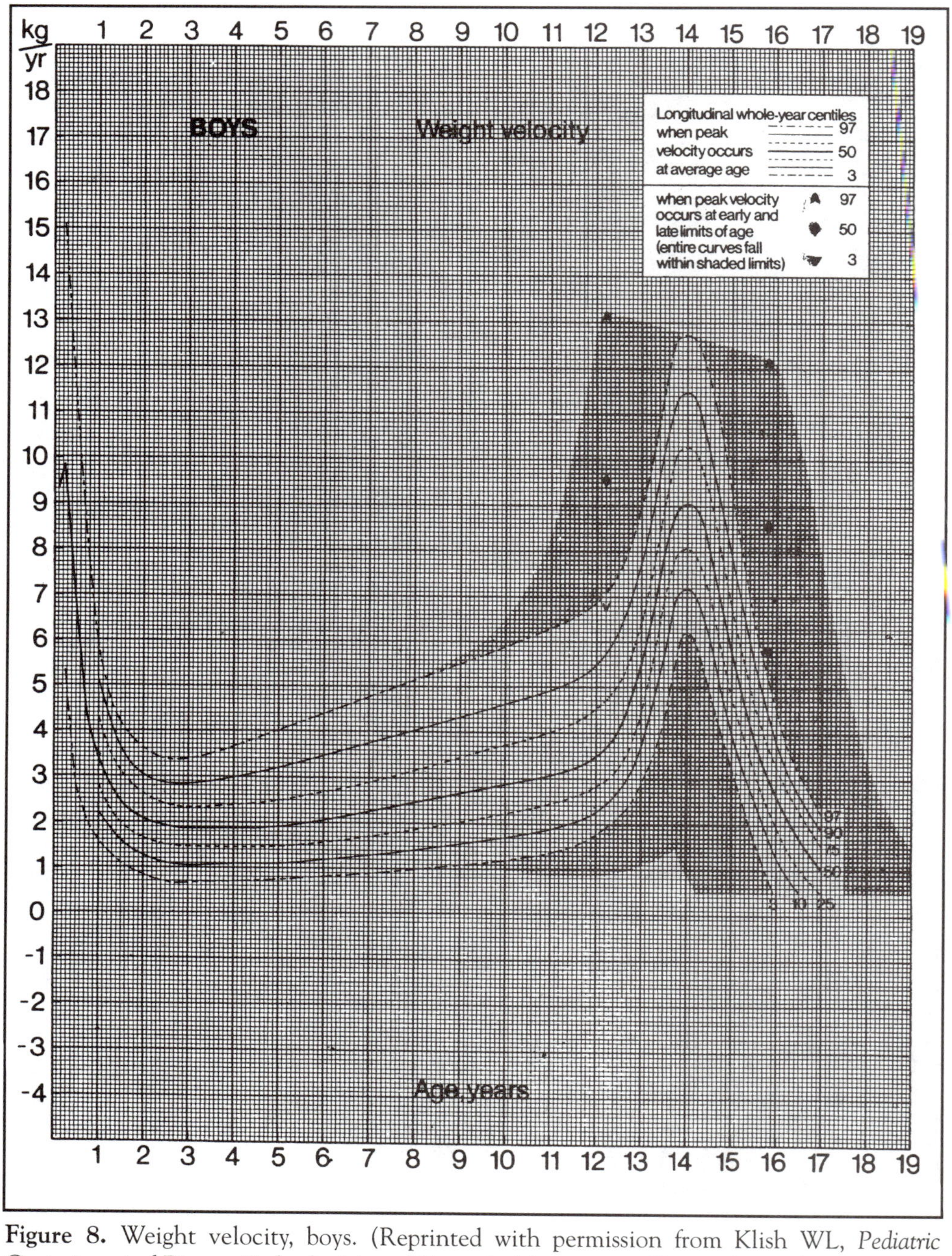

Figure 8. Weight velocity, boys. (Reprinted with permission from Klish WL, *Pediatric Gastrointestinal Disease-Pathophysiology, Diagnosis, Management*, Tanner JM, Whitehouse RH (eds), 1098-1099, copyright 1993, with permission from Elsevier).

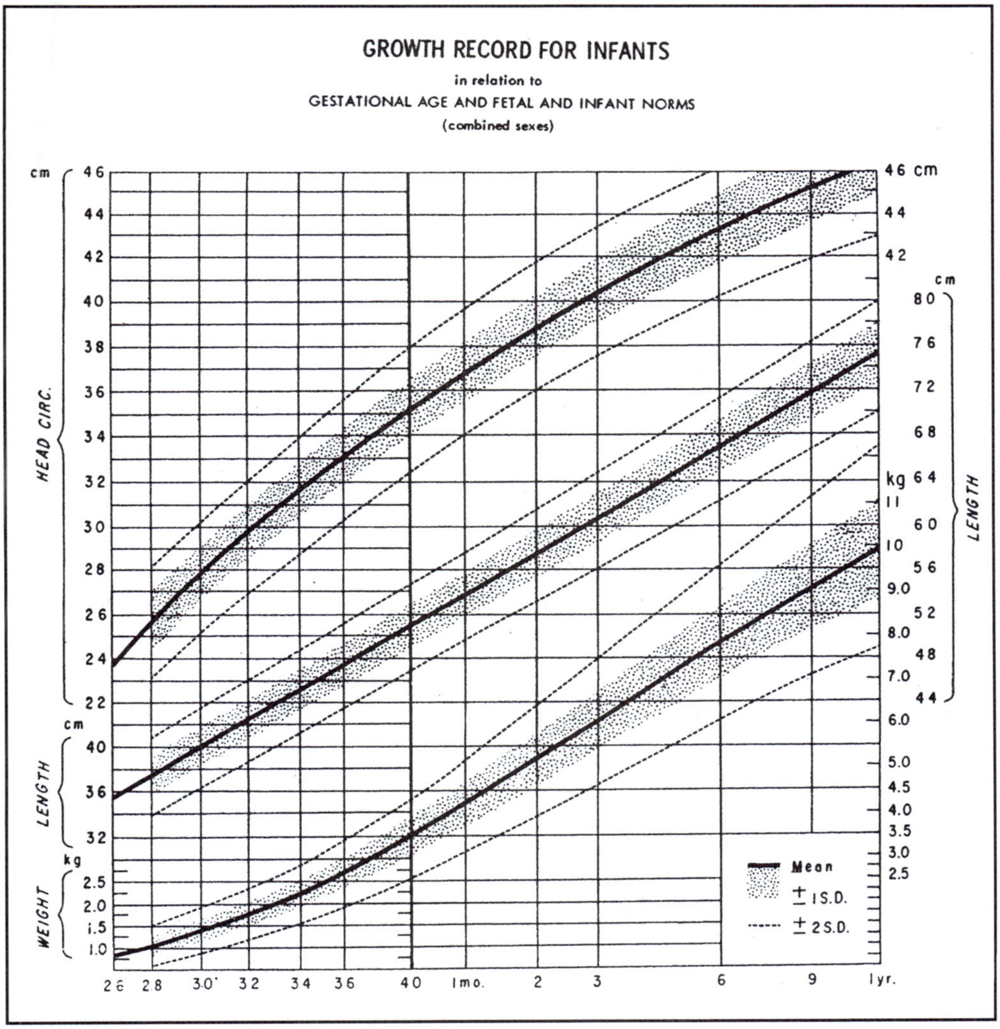

Figure 9. Growth record for infants in relation to gestational age and infant norms. (Reprinted with permission from Babson SG, Benda GI, *J Peds*, Growth graphs for the clinical assessment of infants of varying gestational age, 89, 814-820, copyright 1976, with permission from Elsevier.)

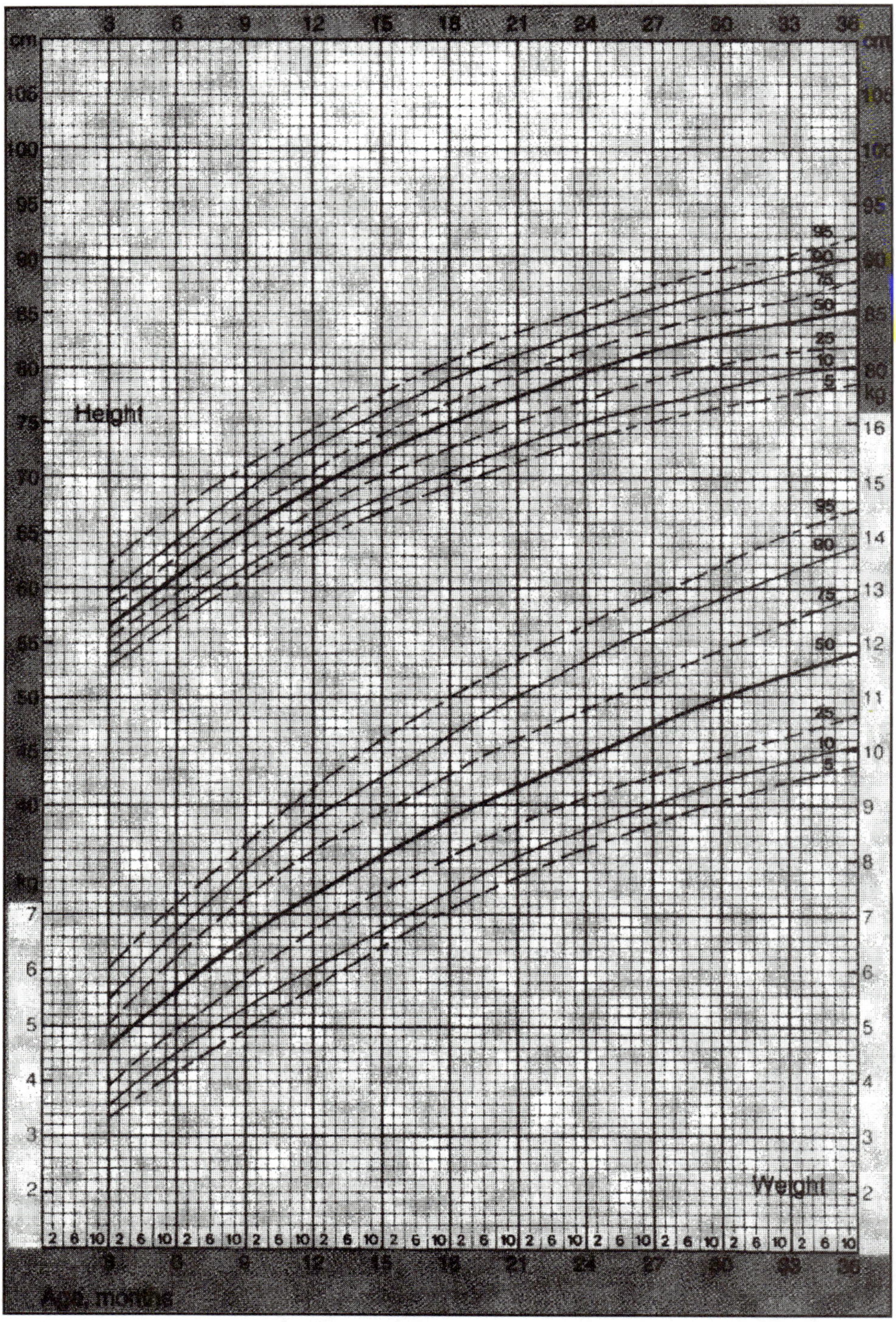

Figure 10. Down syndrome, height and weight for girls, 1 to 36 months. (Reprinted with permission from Cronk C, Crocker AC, Pueschel SM, et al. Growth charts for children with Down syndrome: 1 month to 18 years of age. *Pediatrics*. 1988;81:102-110.)

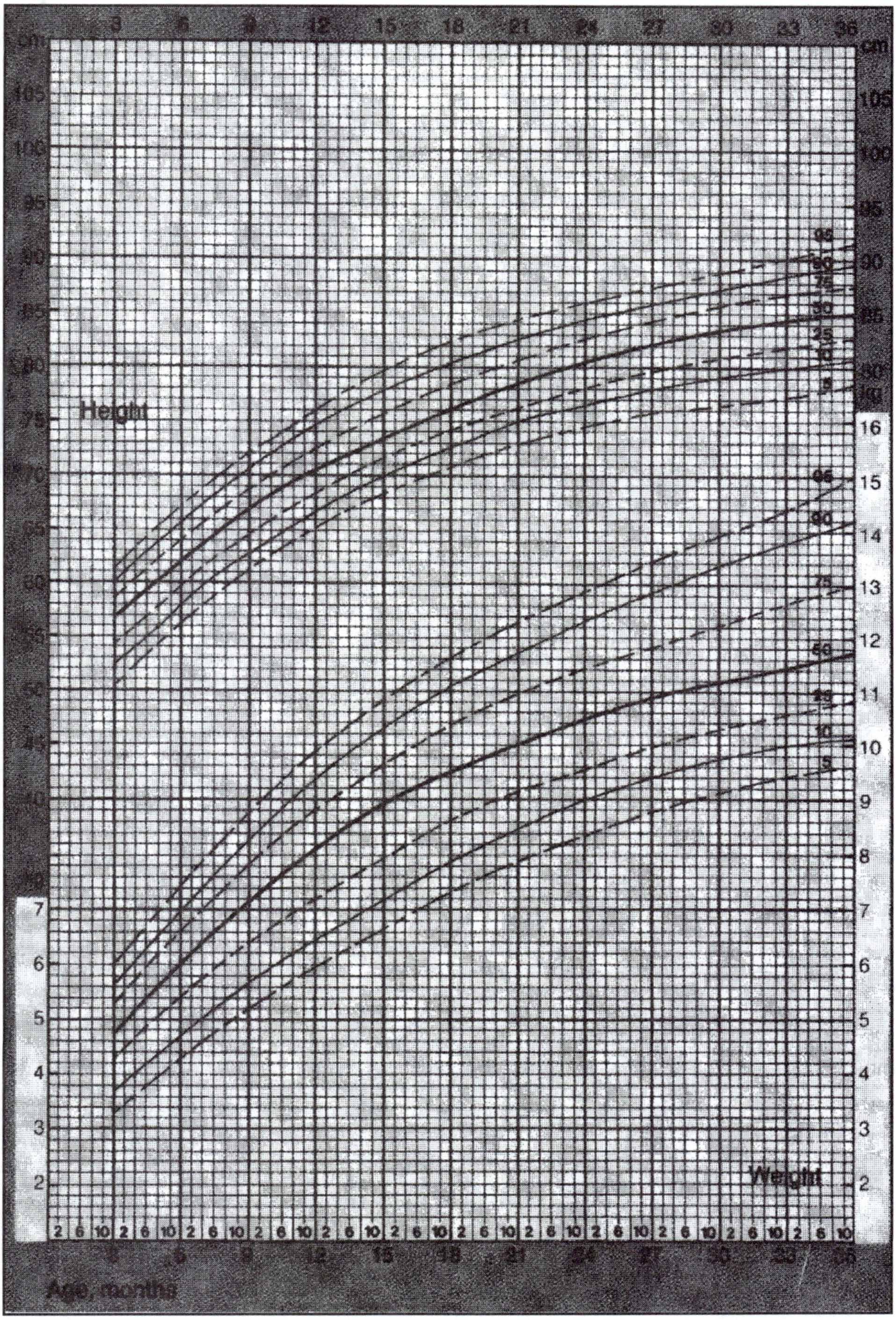

Figure 11. Down syndrome, height and weight for boys, 1 to 36 months. (Reprinted with permission from Cronk C, Crocker AC, Pueschel SM, et al. Growth charts for children with Down syndrome: 1 month to 18 years of age. *Pediatrics*. 1988;81:102-110.)

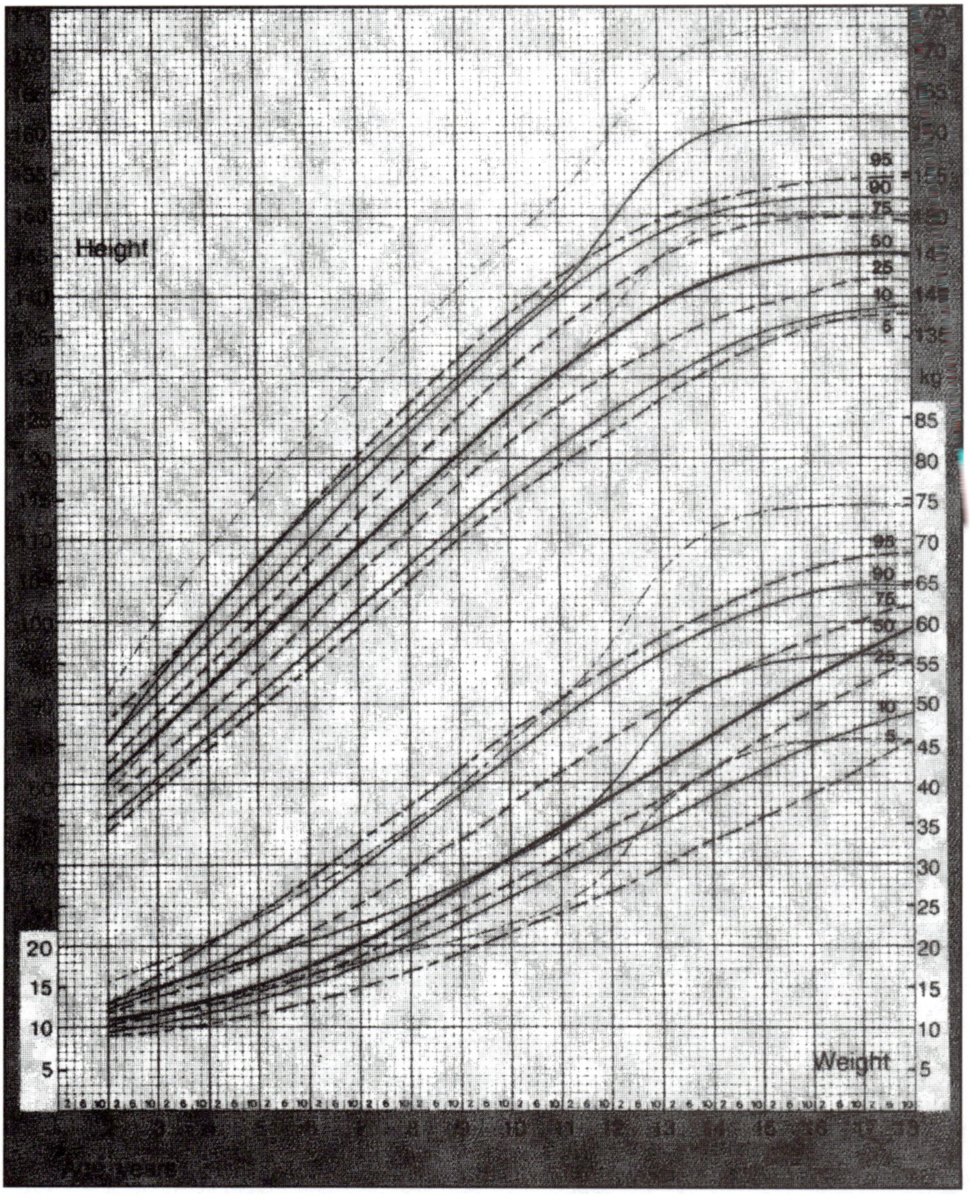

Figure 12. Down syndrome, height and weight for girls, 2 to 18 years. (Reprinted with permission from Cronk C, Crocker AC, Pueschel SM, et al. Growth charts for children with Down syndrome: 1 month to 18 years of age. *Pediatrics*. 1988;81:102-110.)

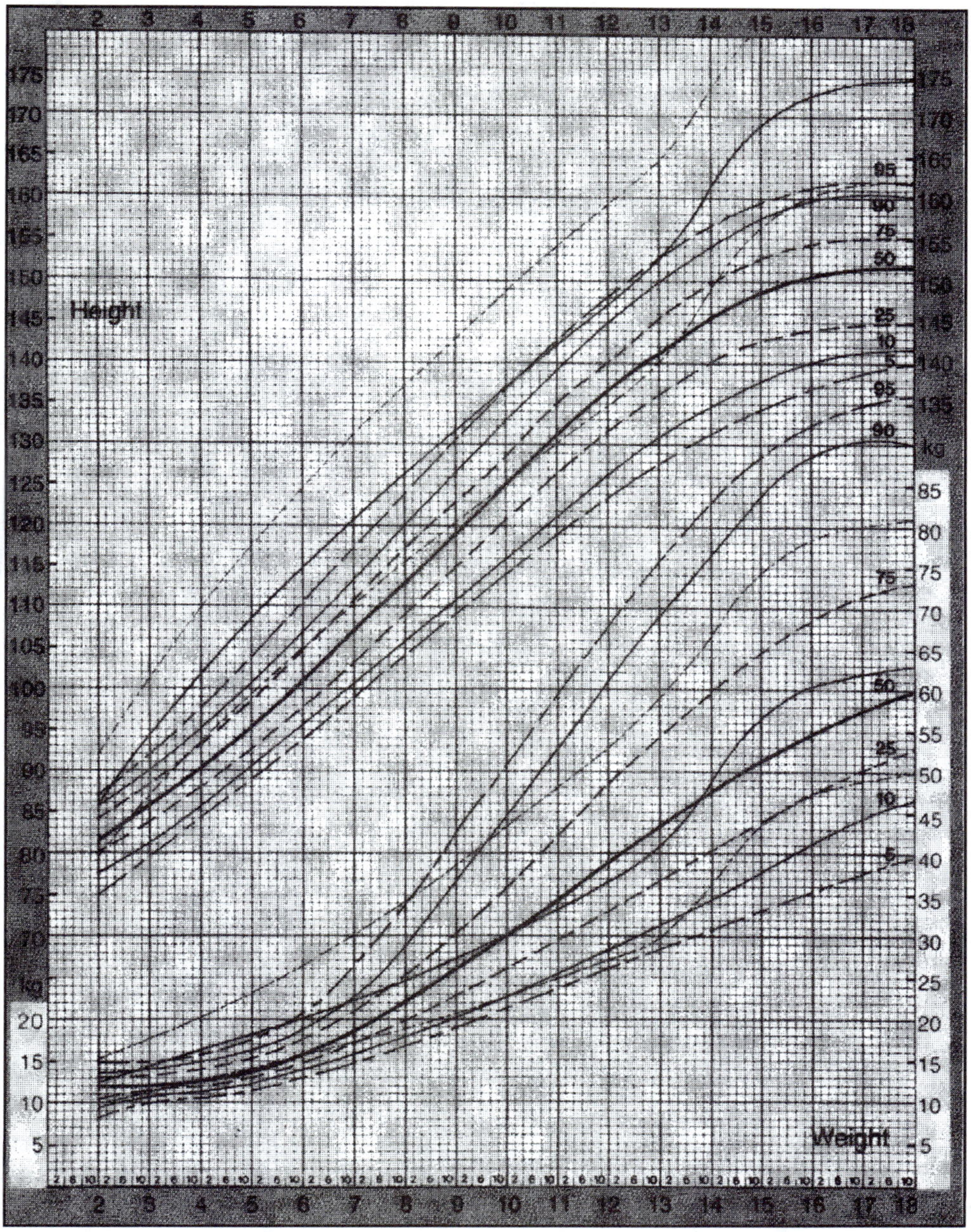

Figure 13. Down syndrome, height and weight for boys, 2 to 18 years. (Reprinted with permission from Cronk C, Crocker AC, Pueschel SM, et al. Growth charts for children with Down syndrome: 1 month to 18 years of age. *Pediatrics*. 1988;81:102-110.)

Birth to 36 months: Girls
Head circumference-for-age and
Weight-for-length percentiles

NAME ______________________

RECORD # ____________

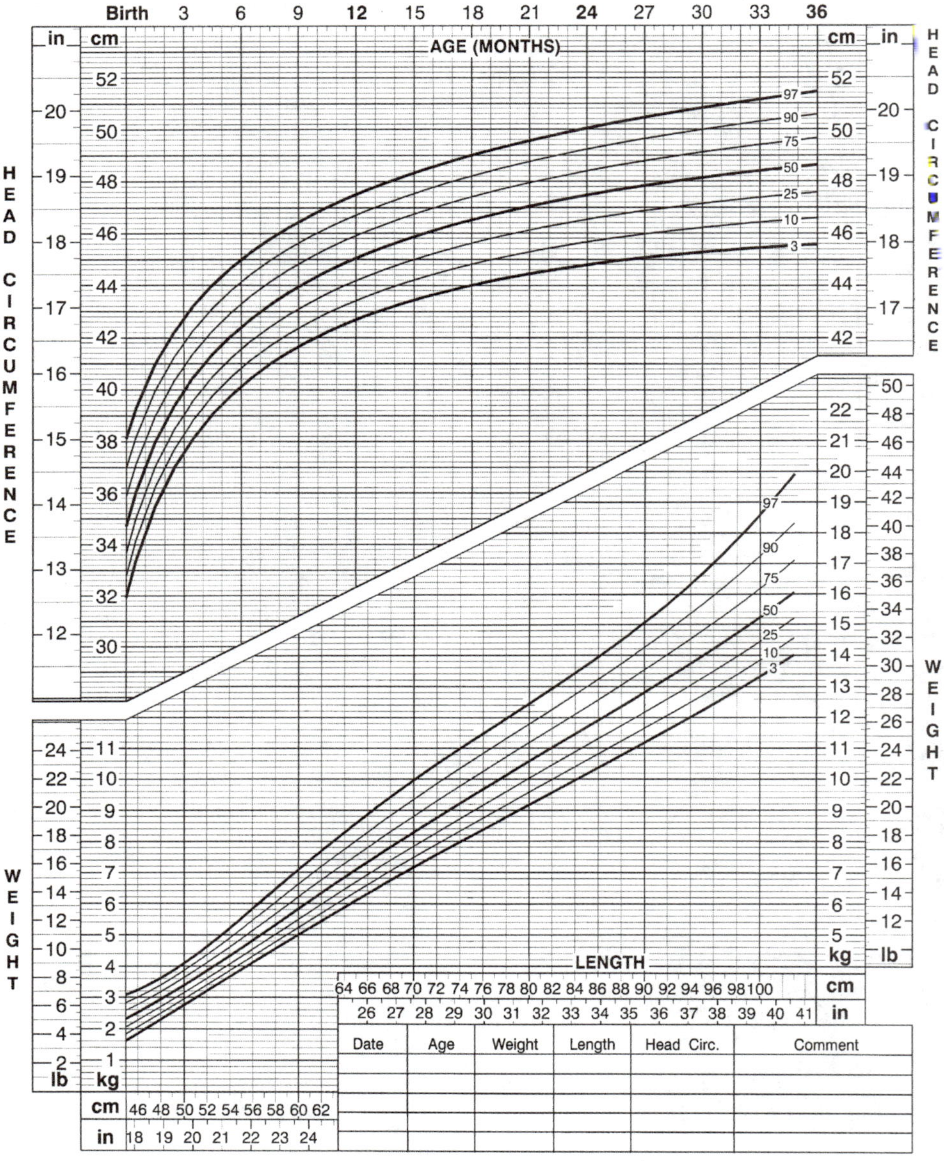

Published May 30, 2000 (modified 10/16/00).
SOURCE: Developed by the National Center for Health Statistics in collaboration with the National Center for Chronic Disease Prevention and Health Promotion (2000).
http://www.cdc.gov/growthcharts

Figure 14. Girls: birth to 36 months head circumference-for-age and weight-for-length NCHS percentiles.

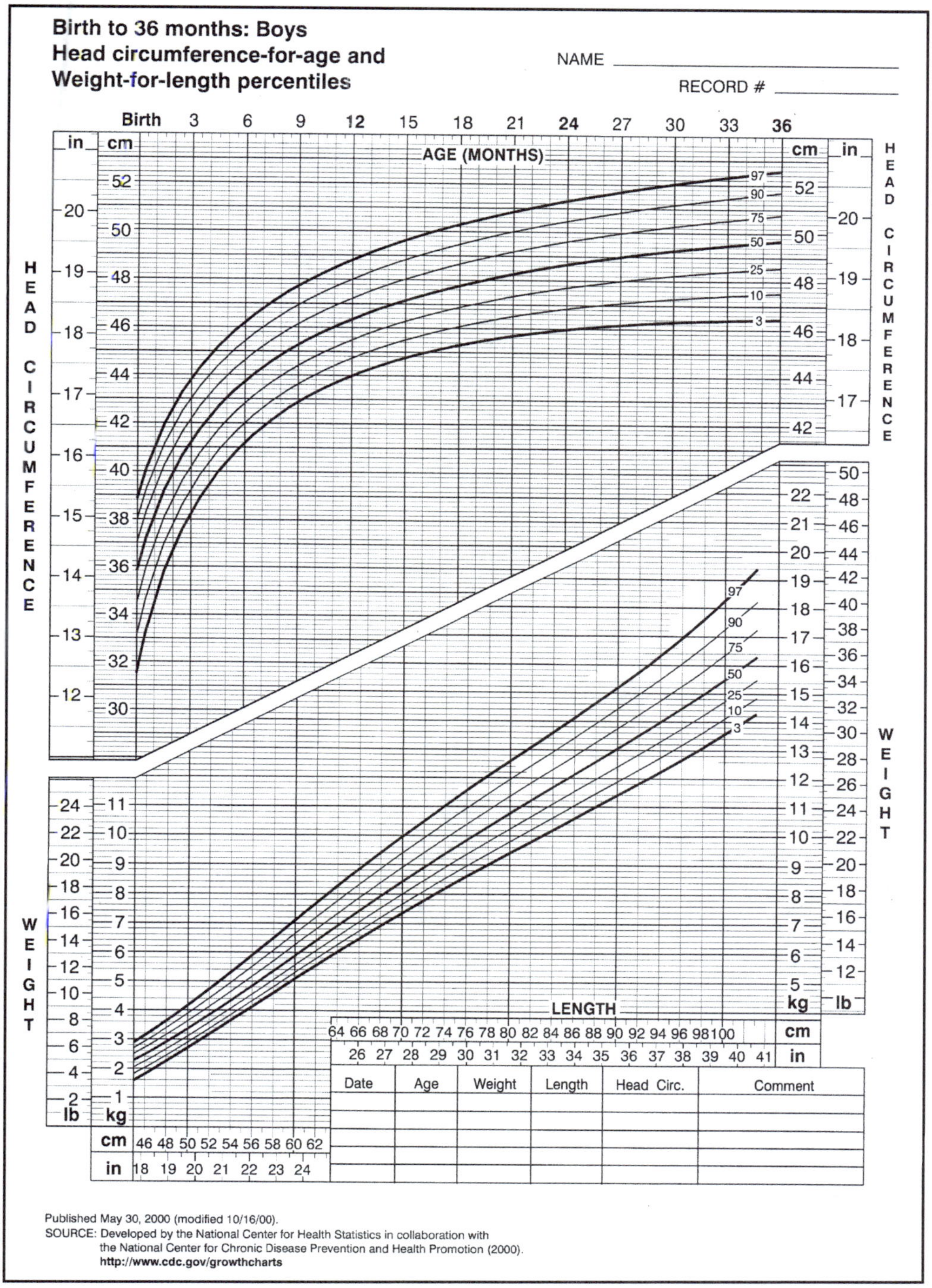

Figure 15. Boys: birth to 36 months head circumference-for-age and weight-for-length NCHS percentiles.

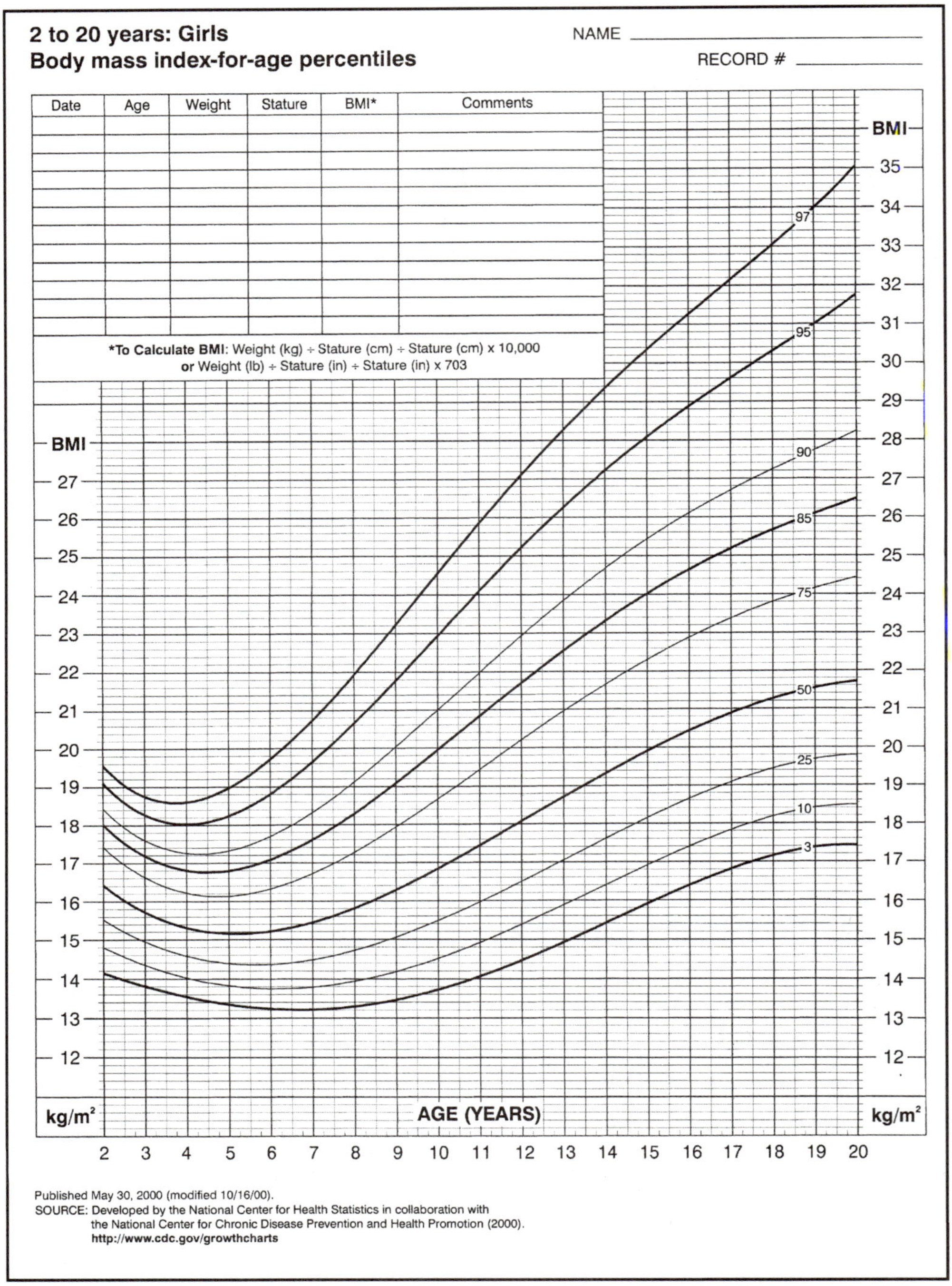

Figure 16. Girls: 2 to 20 years body mass index-for-age NCHS percentiles.

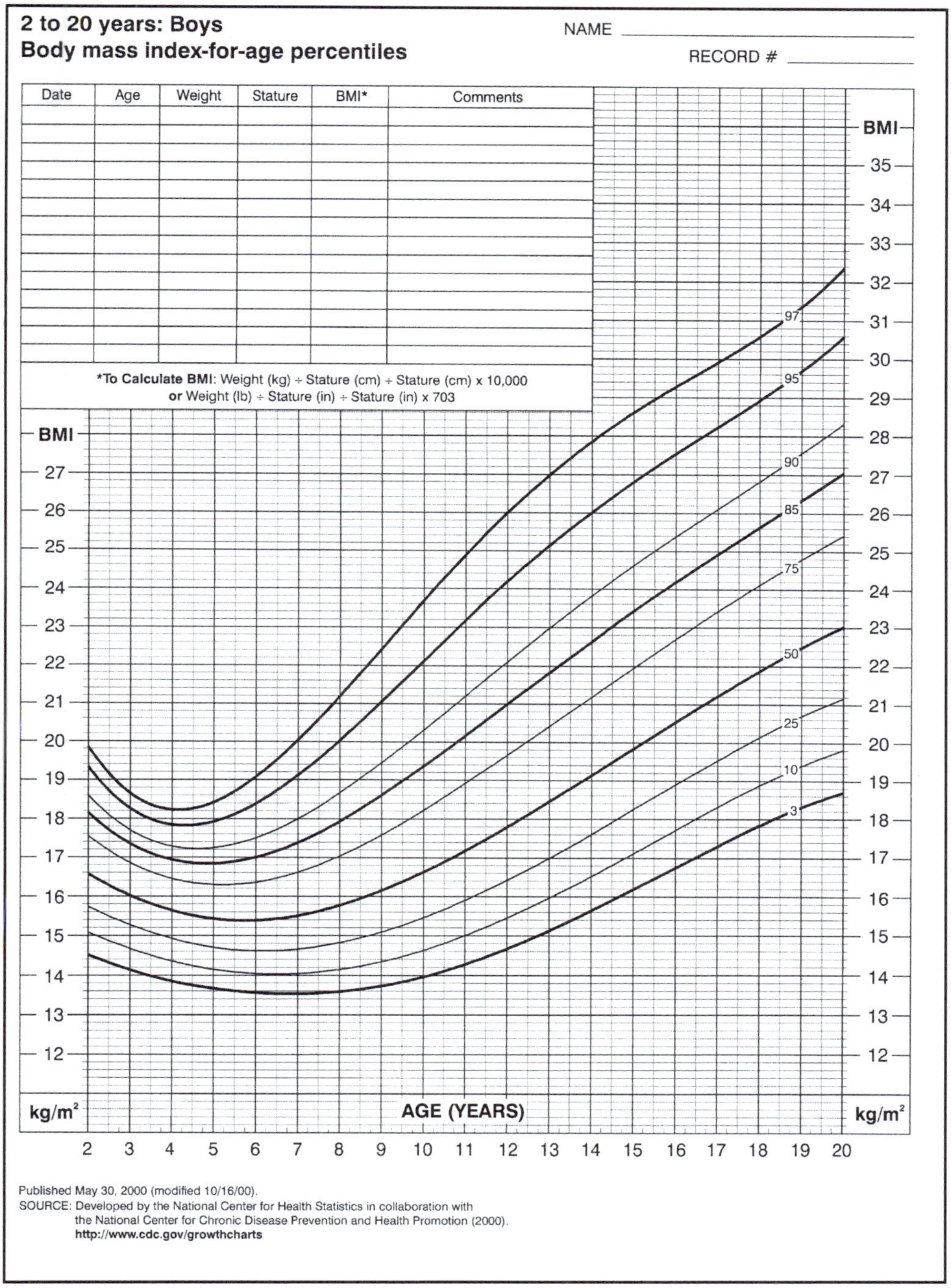

Figure 17. Boys: 2 to 20 years body mass index-for-age NCHS percentiles.

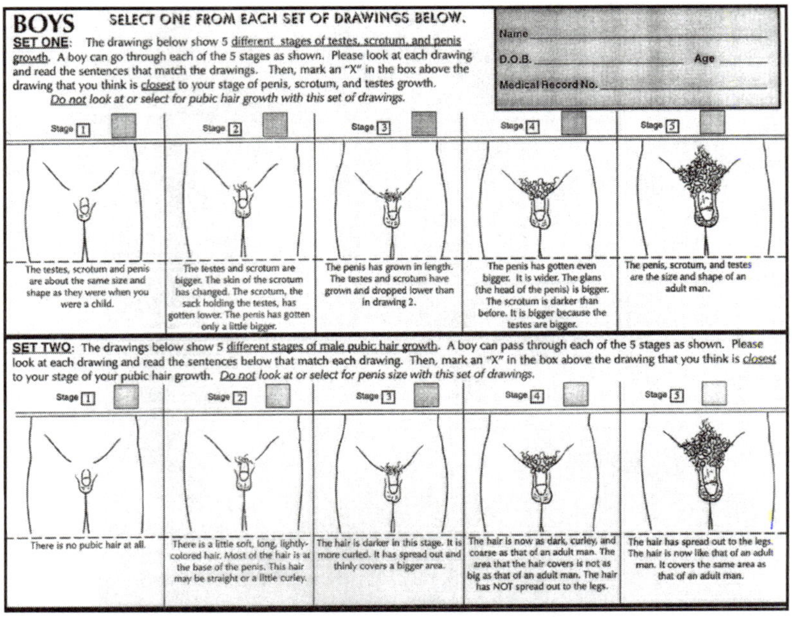

Figure 18. Male pubertal assessment. (Reprinted with permission from *Journal of Youth and Adolescence*. 1993;9(3): 271-280, Plenum.)

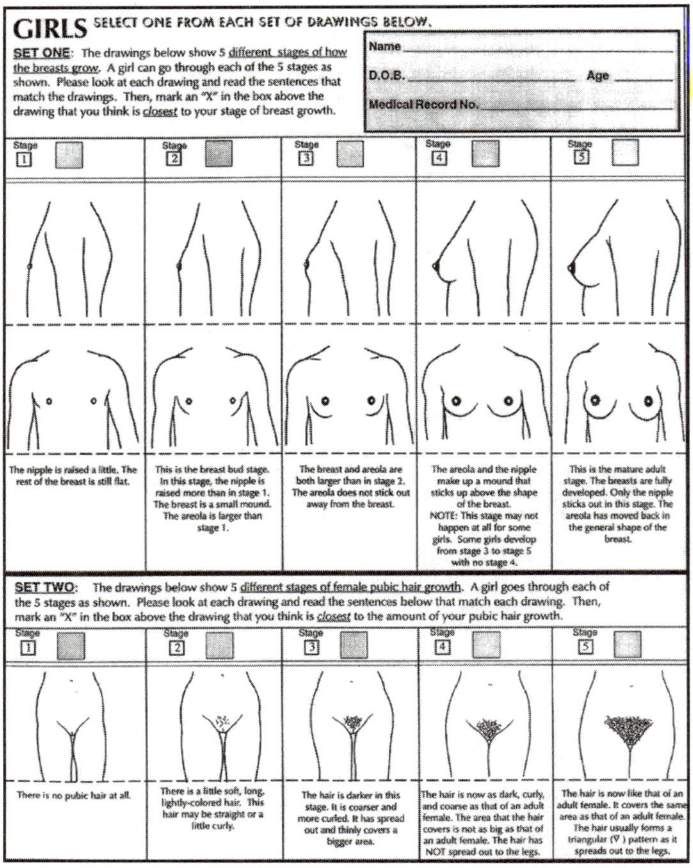

Figure 19. Female pubertal assessment. (Reprinted with permission from *Journal of Youth and Adolescence*. 1993;9(3): 271-280, Plenum.)

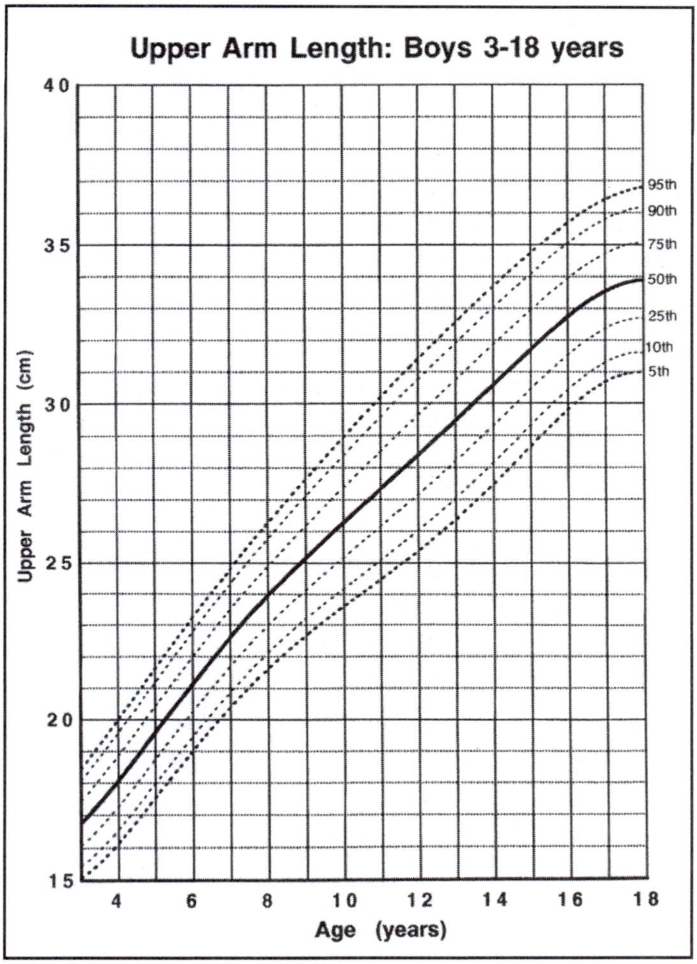

Figure 20. Upper arm length: boys 3 to 18 years. Reprinted with permission from Stallings VA, Zemel BS. Nutritional assessment of the disabled child. In: Sullivan P, Rosenbloom L, eds. *Clinics in Developmental Medicine: Feeding the Disabled Child.* London: MacKeith Press; 1996;62-76.

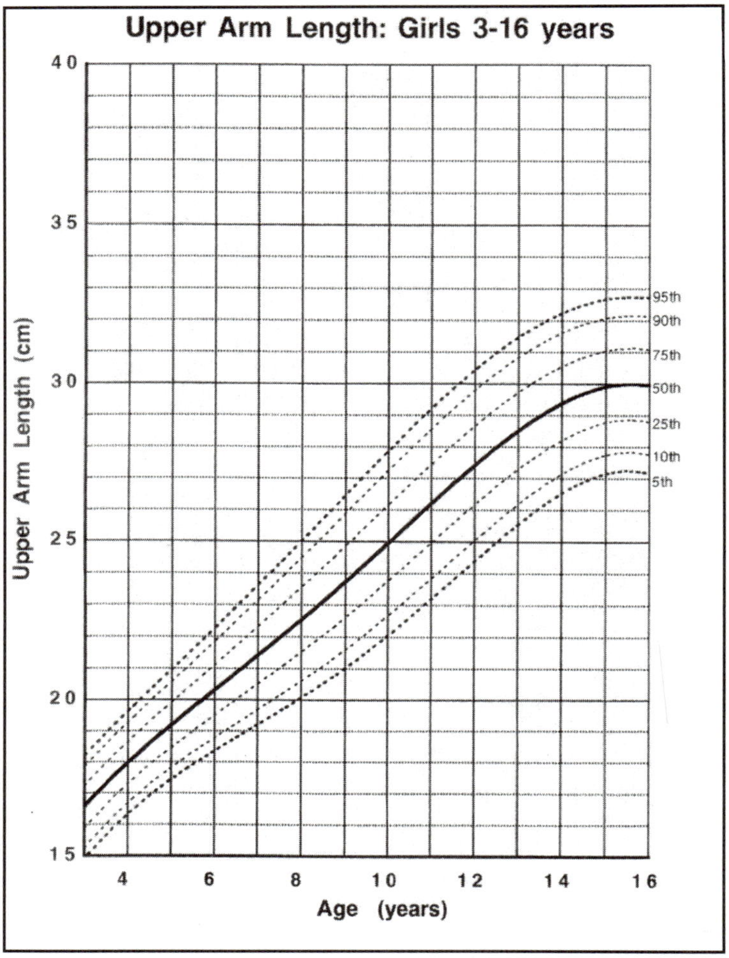

Figure 21. Upper arm length: girls 3 to 16 years. Reprinted with permission from Stallings VA, Zemel BS. Nutritional assessment of the disabled child. In: Sullivan P, Rosenbloom L, eds. *Clinics in Developmental Medicine: Feeding the Disabled Child.* London: MacKeith Press; 1996;62-76.

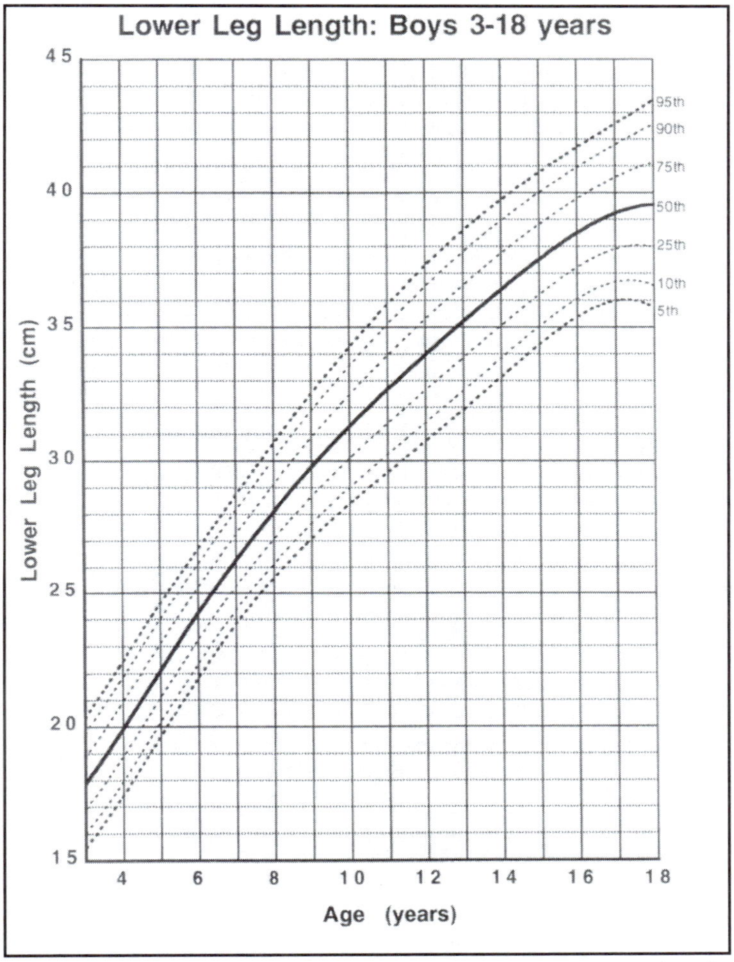

Figure 22. Lower leg length: boys 3 to 18 years. Reprinted with permission from Stallings VA, Zemel BS. Nutritional assessment of the disabled child. In: Sullivan P, Rosenbloom L, eds. *Clinics in Developmental Medicine: Feeding the Disabled Child.* London: MacKeith Press; 1996;62-76.

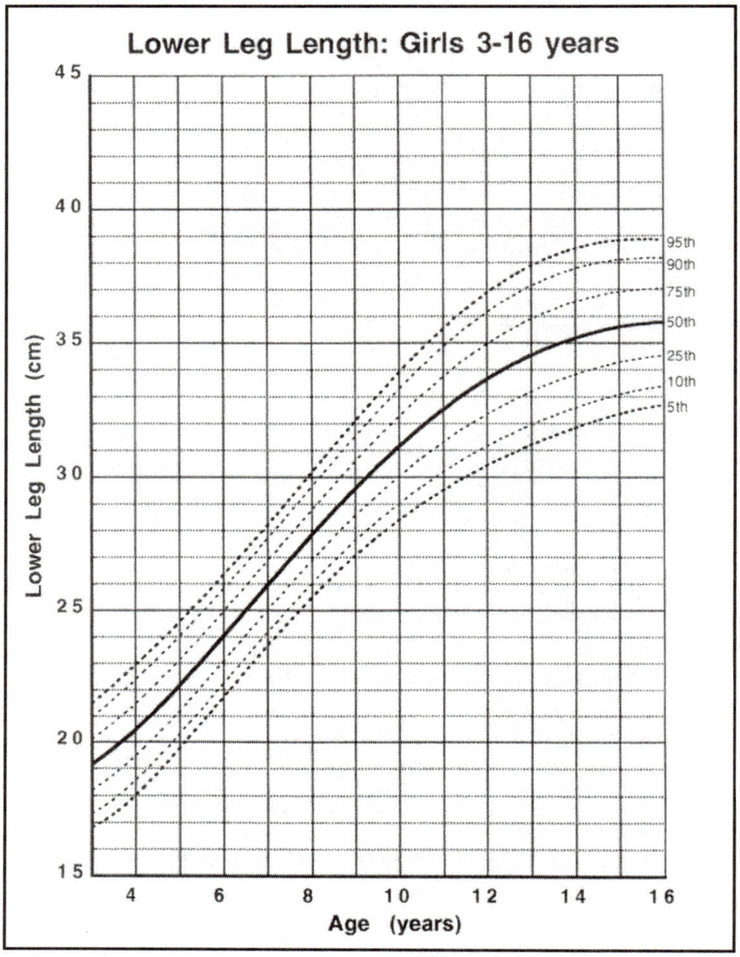

Figure 23. Lower leg length: girls 3 to 16 years. Reprinted with permission from Stallings VA, Zemel BS. Nutritional assessment of the disabled child. In: Sullivan P, Rosenbloom L, eds. *Clinics in Developmental Medicine: Feeding the Disabled Child.* London: MacKeith Press; 1996;62-76.

Appendix C

Pediatric Tables

TABLE 1

Etiology of Malnutrition

Mechanism	Disorders
Non-Organic	
Psychosocial	Poor maternal-child interactions, poor feeding technique, psychologically disturbed mother, unusual maternal nutritional beliefs, errors in formula preparation, emotional deprivation, dwarfism, child neglect, anorexia, bulimia
Organic	
Inability to suck, swallow, or masticate	CNS pathology (psychomotor retardation), neuromuscular disease (Werdnig-Hoffman, myotonia congenita, dysautonomia)
Maldigestion, malabsorption	Cystic Fibrosis, celiac disease, Shwachman-Diamond syndrome, chronic diarrhea, intestinal resection (short-gut syndrome), chronic cholestatic liver disease, HIV
Increased requirements	Intrauterine growth retardation, small for gestation age, prematurity, critical illness, catch-up growth
Poor nutrient utilization	Renal failure, renal tubular acidosis, inborn errors of metabolism
Vomiting	CNS abnormality (tumor, infection, increased pressure), metabolic toxin (inborn errors of amino or organic acid metabolism), intestinal obstruction (pyloric stenosis, malrotation), renal tubular disease
Regurgitation	Gastroesophageal reflux, eosinophilic esophagitis, hiatus hernia, rumination syndrome
Elevated metabolic rate ± Anorexia	Thyrotoxicosis, chronic disease (bronchopulmonary dysplasia, heart failure), cancer, inflammatory lesions (SLE, Crohn's disease, chronic infection eg, TB), immunodeficiency diseases, burns
Reduced growth potential	Chromosomal disorders, primordial dwarfism, skeletal dysplasia, specific syndromes (fetal alcohol)
Obesity	Prader Willi, polycystic ovary syndrome, hypothyroidism, pseudohypoparathyroidism, Cushing syndrome, Turner syndrome, Hyperinsulinemia

TABLE 2

Upper Arm Muscle Area in Children Aged 1 to Adulthood

Age Group, yrs	Arm Muscle Area Percentiles (mm²) 5th	10th	25th	50th	75th	90th	95th
Males							
1 to 1.9	956	1014	1133	1278	1447	1644	1720
2 to 2.9	973	1040	1190	1345	1557	1690	1787
3 to 3.9	1095	1201	1357	1484	1618	1750	1853
4 to 4.9	1207	1264	1408	1579	1747	1926	2008
5 to 5.9	1298	1411	1550	1720	1884	2089	2285
6 to 6.9	1360	1447	1605	1815	2056	2297	2493
7 to 7.9	1497	1548	1808	2027	2246	2494	2886
8 to 8.9	1550	1664	1895	2089	2296	2628	2788
9 to 9.9	1811	1884	2067	2288	2657	3053	3257
10 to 10.9	1930	2027	2182	2575	2903	3486	3882
11 to 11.9	2016	2156	2382	2670	3022	3359	4225
12 to 12.9	2216	2339	2649	3022	3496	3968	4640
13 to 13.9	2363	2546	3044	3553	4081	4502	4794
14 to 14.9	2830	3147	3586	3963	4575	5368	5530
15 to 15.9	3138	3317	3788	4481	5134	5631	5900
16 to 16.9	3625	4044	4352	4951	5753	6576	6980
17 to 17.9	3998	4252	4777	5286	5950	6886	7726
18 to 18.9	4070	4481	5066	5552	6374	7067	8355
19 to 24.9	4508	4777	5274	5913	6660	7606	8200
Females							
1 to 1.9	885	973	1084	1221	1378	1535	1627
2 to 2.9	973	1029	1119	1269	1405	1595	1727
3 to 3.9	1014	1133	1227	1396	1563	1690	1846
4 to 4.9	1058	1171	1313	1475	1644	1832	1958
5 to 5.9	1238	1301	1423	1598	1825	2012	2159
6 to 6.9	1354	1414	1513	1683	1877	2182	2323
7 to 7.9	1330	1441	1602	1815	2045	2332	2469
8 to 8.9	1513	1566	1808	2034	2327	2657	2996
9 to 9.9	1723	1788	1976	2227	2571	2987	3112
10 to 10.9	1740	1784	2019	2296	2583	2873	3093
11 to 11.9	1784	1987	2316	2612	3071	3739	3953
12 to 12.9	2092	2182	2579	2904	3225	3655	3847
13 to 13.9	2269	2426	2657	3130	3529	4081	4568
14 to 14.9	2418	2562	2874	3220	3704	4294	4850
15 to 15.9	2426	2518	2847	3248	3689	4123	4756
16 to 16.9	2308	2567	2865	3248	3718	4353	4946
17 to 17.9	2442	2674	2996	3336	3883	4552	5251
18 to 18.9	2398	2538	2917	3243	3694	4461	4767
19 to 24.9	2538	2728	3026	3406	3877	4439	4940

Adapted from Frisancho AR. New norms of upper limb fat and muscle areas for assessment of nutritional status. *Am J Clin Nutr*. 1981;34:2540-45.

Table 3

Standard Milk-Based Infant Formulas

Product (Manufacturer)	Human Milk	Enfamil W/Iron* (Mead Johnson)	Enfamil 24 (Mead Johnson)	Enfamil AR (Mead Johnson)	Enfamil Lacto-Free(Mead Johnson)	Enfamil Lipil (Mead Johnson)	Good Start (Nestle)	SimilacW/ Iron* (Ross)
Calories/100 ml	72 + 5	67	80.6	67	68	67	67	67.5
Protein gm/100ml	1.0	1.4	1.8	1.6	1.4	1.4	1.6	1.4
Protein source	60%whey 40% casein	60% whey 40% casein	Whey &nonfat milk	18% whey 82% casein	20% whey 80% casein	Nonfat milk & whey protein concentrate	100% whey	18% whey 82% casein
CHO gm/100ml	7.2+0.25	7.3	8.8	7.3	7.4	7.3	7.3	7.3
CHO source	lactose	lactose	lactose	lactose, rice starch & maltodextrin	corn syrup solids	lactose	lactose, corn maltodextrin	lactose
Fat gm/100ml	3.9+0.4	3.5	4.3	3.4	3.6	3.5	3.4	3.65
Fat source	Human milk	Palm olein, soy, coconut, & high-oleic safflower oils (45:20:20:15)	Palm olein, soy, coconut, & high-oleic sunflower oils	Palm olein, soy, coconut & high-oleic safflower oils (45:20:20:15)	Palm olein,soy, coconut, &high-oleic safflower oils (45:20:20:15)	Palm olein, soy, coconut, high-oleic sunflower & soy lecithin oils. <1% M. alpina & C. cohnii oil*	Palm olein, soy, coconut, & high-oleic safflower oils (47:26:21:6)	High-oleic safflower, coconut, & soy oils (40:30:30)
Osmolality mOsm/kg	290±5	300	360	230	200	300	265	300
Sodium mEq (mg)/100ml	.7 (17.9)	.78 (18)	1.0 (22)	1.1 (26)	.9 (20)	.78 (18)	.69 (16)	0.67 (16.2)
Potassium mEq (mg)/100ml	1.3 (52.8)	1.8 (72)	2.3 (88)	1.8 (72)	1.9 (74)	1.8 (72)	1.6 (65)	1.8 (71)
Calcium mEq (mg)/100ml	1.5 (28)	2.6 (52)	3.2 (63)	2.6 (52)	2.7 (54)	2.6 (52)	2.1 (42)	2.6 (53)
Phosphorus mEq(mg)/100ml	.9 (14)	2.2 (35)	2.7 (43)	2.2 (35)	2.3 (36)	2.2 (35)	1.5 (24)	1.8 (28)
Iron mg/100ml	.03	1.2 *low iron formula=.7	1.2	1.2	1.2	1.2	1.0	1.2 *low iron formula =.5
Notes:			RTF available hospital use only. Prepare from concentrate for home use.			*C. cohnii source of DHA M. alpina source of ARA		

TABLE 3 CONTINUED

Standard Milk-Based Infant Formulas

Product (Manufacturer)	Similac 24 (Ross)	Similac Advance (Ross)	Similac Lacto-free (Ross)
Calories/100 ml	80.6	67.5	67
Protein gm/100ml	2.1	1.4	1.4
Protein source	Nonfat milk	Nonfat milk & whey protein concentrate	Milk protein isolate
CHO gm/100ml	8.4	7.3	7.1
CHO source	Lactose	Lactose	Corn syrup solids & sucrose (55:45)
Fat gm/100ml	4.2	3.6	3.6
Fat source	Soy & coconut oils	High-oleic safflower, soy & coconut oils (.15%DHA & .4%ARA)*	Soy & coconut oils (60:40)
Osmolality mOsm/kg	380	300	200
Sodium mEq (mg)/100ml	1.19 (27)	.67 (16)	.8 (20)
Potassium mEq (mg)/100ml	2.7 (106)	1.8 (70)	1.8 (71)
Calcium mEq (mg)/100ml	3.6 (72)	2.6 (52)	2.8 (56)
Phosphorus mEq(mg)/100ml	3.6 (56)	1.8 (28)	2.4 (37)
Iron mg/100ml	1.4	1.2	1.2
Notes:	RTF available for hospital use only. Prepare from concentrate for home use.	*C. cohnii source of DHA M. alpina source of ARA	

TABLE 4

Standard Soy-Based Formulas

Product (Manufacturer)	Alsoy (Nestle)	Isomil (Ross)	Isomil DF (Ross)	Isomil SF (Ross)	Prosobee (Mead Johnson)
Calories/100 ml	67	67	67	67	67
Protein gm/100ml	1.8	1.6	1.7	1.8	1.6
Protein source	Soy protein isolate	Soy protein isolate	Soyprotein isolate w/fiber	Soyprotein isolate	Soy protein isolate
CHO gm/100ml	7.4	6.8	6.7	6.7	7.0
CHO source	Corn malto-dextrin & sucrose	Corn syrup & sucrose (80:20)	Corn syrup & Sucrose (60:40)	Hydrolyzed corn starch	Corn syrup solids
Fat gm/100ml	3.3	3.6	3.6	3.6	3.5
Fat source	Palm olein, soy, coco-nut, & high-oleic safflower oils (47:26:21:6)	High-oleic safflower, coconut, & soy oils (40:30:30)	Soy & coconut oils (60:40)	Soy & coconut oils (60:40)	Palm olein, soy, coconut, & high-oleic sunflower oils (45:20:20:15)
Osmolality mOsm/kg	200	200	240	180	200
Sodium mEq (mg)/100ml	.9 (22)	1.2 (29)	.9 (22)	1.3 (29)	1.0 (24)
Potassium mEq (mg)/100ml	1.9 (77)	1.8 (72)	1.9 (77)	1.9 (77)	2.0 (80)
Calcium mEq (mg)/100ml	3.5 (70)	3.4 (70)	3.5 (70)	3.5 (70)	3.4 (70)
Phosphorus mEq(mg)/100ml	2.6 (40)	3.3 (50)	2.6 (40)	3.2 (50)	2.7 (55)
Iron mg/100ml	1.2	1.2	1.2	1.2	1.2

Notes:

TABLE 5

Formulas for Preterm Infants: Designed for Rapidly Growing LBW Infants

Product (Manufacturer)	Preterm Human Milk	Enfamil Human Milk Fortifier (Mead Johnson)	Similac Human Milk Fortifier (Ross)	Enfamil Premature W/iron 20* (Mead Johnson)	Enfamil Premature W/iron 24 (Mead Johnson)	Similac Special Care W/iron 20* (Ross)	Similac Special Care W/iron 24 (Ross)
Calories/100 ml	67	14	14	67	80	67	81
Protein gm/100ml	1.4	1.1	1.0	2.0	2.3	1.8	2.1
Protein source	Preterm human milk	Whey protein concentrate & casein (60:40)	Nonfat milk & whey protein concentrate	Nonfat milk & whey protein concentrate (60:40)	Nonfat milk & whey protein concentrate (60:40)	Nonfat milk & whey protein concentrate	Nonfat milk & whey protein concentrate
CHO gm/100ml	6.6	1.1	1.8	7.4	8.8	7.0	8.5
CHO source	lactose	Corn syrup solids & lactose	Corn syrup solids	Corn syrup solids & lactose (60:40)	Corn syrup solids & lactose (60:40)	Corn syrup solids & lactose (50:50)	Corn syrup solids & lactose (50:50)
Fat gm/100ml	3.8	.65	.36	3.4	4.0	3.6	4.3
Fat source	Preterm human milk	20% MCT	MCT & soy, lecithin oils	MCT, soy, & coconut oils (40:40:20)	MCT, soy, & coconut oils (40:40:20)	MCT, soy, & coconut oils (50:30:20)	MCT, soy, & coconut oils (50:30:20)
Osmolality mOsm/kg	290	63	90	260	310	235	280
Sodium mEq (mg)/100ml	1.0 (24)	.47 (11)	.65 (15)	1.1 (26)	1.3 (30)	1.2 (28)	1.5 (34)
Potassium mEq (mg)/100ml	1.4 (56)	.5 (20)	1.6 (63)	1.7 (68)	2.0 (81)	2.2 (86)	2.6 (104)
Calcium mEq (mg)/100ml	1.2 (24)	4.5 (90)	5.8 (117)	5.5 (110)	6.5 (130)	6 (120)	7.2 (145)
Phosphorus mEq(mg)/100ml	.8 (12)	2.9 (45)	4.3 (63)	3.5 (55)	4.2 (65)	4.3 (66)	5.2 (80)
Iron mg/100ml	.12	1.4	.35	1.2 *low iron=.16	1.4	1.2 *low iron=.2	1.4
Notes:		4 packets of fortifier (.81g/pkt)	4 packets of fortifier (.9g/pkt)				

TABLE 5 CONTINUED

Formulas for Preterm Infants: Post-Discharge Through the First Year of Life

Product (Manufacturer)	Enfamil EnfaCare (Mead Johnson)	Similac NeoSure (Ross)
Calories/100 ml	74	74
Protein gm/100ml	2.0	1.9
Protein source	Whey & nonfat milk protein concentrate (60:40)	Whey & nonfat milk protein concentrate
CHO gm/100ml	7.9	7.6
CHO source	Corn syrup solids & lactose (60:40)	Maltodextrin & lactose (50:50)
Fat gm/100ml	3.9	4.1
Fat source	High-oleic sunflower, soy, MCT, & coconut oils (35:30:20:15)	Soy, coconut, & MCT oils (45:30:25)
Osmolality mOsm/kg	260	250
Sodium mEq (mg)/100ml	1.1 (25)	1.0 (24)
Potassium mEq (mg)/100ml	1.9 (77)	2.6 (105)
Calcium mEq (mg)/100ml	4.4 (88)	3.8 (78)
Phosphorus mEq(mg)/100ml	3.1 (48)	1.1 (46)
Iron mg/100ml	1.2	1.2

Notes:

TABLE 6

Specialized Formulas for Infants

	Formulas with Low Molecular Weight Peptides or Amino Acids					Low in LCF	Low in Electrolytes & Minerals
Product (Manufacturer)	Alimentum (Ross)	Neocate (SHS)	Nutramigen (Mead Johnson)	Pregestimil (Mead Johnson)	Pregestimil 24 (Mead Johnson)	Portagen (Mead Johnson)	Similac PM 60/40 (Ross)
Calories/100 ml	67	67	67	67	81	67	67
Protein gm/100ml	1.8	2.0	1.8	1.8	2.2	2.3	1.4
Protein source	Hydrolyzed casein w/added L-cystine, L-tyrosine & L-tryptophan	L-amino acids	Hydrolyzed casein w/added L-cystine L-tryosine & L-tryptophan	Hydrolyzed casein w/added L-cystine, L-tyrosine & L-tryptophan	Hydrolyzed casein w/added L-cystine, L-tyrosine & L-tryptophan	Sodium caseinate	Whey Protein concentrate & sodium caseinate
CHO gm/100ml	6.8	7.8	7.3	6.8	8.0	7.6	6.8
CHO source	Sucrose & modified tapioca starch (70:30)	Corn syrup solids	Corn syrup solids & modified corn starch	Corn syrup solids, dextrose, & modified corn starch	Corn syrup solids, dextrose, & modified corn starch	Corn syrup solids & sucrose	lactose
Fat gm/100ml	3.6	3.0	3.3	3.7	4.4	3.2	3.7
Fat source	MCT, soy, & safflower oils (39:33:28)	Refined vegetable, hybrid safflower, coconut, & soy oils	Palm olein, soy, coconut, & high oleic sunflower oils (45:20:20:15)	MCT, soy, corn, & high-oleic safflower oils (55:25:10:10)	MCT, soy, corn & high-oleic safflower oils (55:25:10:10)	MCT & corn oils (86% MCT)	Corn, coconut, & soy oils (50:38:12)
Osmolality mOsm/kg	370	353	320	320	380	230	280
Sodium mEq (mg)/100ml	1.2 (29)	1.0 (24)	1.3 (31)	1.3 (31)	1.6 (37)	1.5 (36)	.67 (16.2)
Potassium mEq (mg)/100ml	2.0 (78)	2.6 (103)	1.8 (73)	1.8 (73)	2.2 (87)	2.1 (83)	1.4 (54)
Calcium mEq (mg)/100ml	3.5 (70)	4.1 (82)	3.1 (62)	3.8 (76)	4.5 (91)	3.1 (62)	1.8 (37)
Phosphorus mEq(mg)/100ml	3.2 (50)	4.0 (62)	2.7 (42)	3.2 (50)	3.8 (59)	3.0 (46)	1.2 (18)
Iron mg/100ml	1.2	1.2	1.2	1.2	1.4	1.2	.47
Notes:				RTF hospital use only. Prepare from powder for home use.	For increased caloric demands and/or fluid restriction. RTF hospital use only. Prepare from powder for home use.	For infants or children with impaired long-chain fat digestion/absorption	For infants whose renal or cardio-vascular system would benefit from lower mineral levels.

TABLE 6 CONTINUED

Specialized Formulas for Infants

	Low LCT	Protein Hydrolysate: High MCT			
Product (Manufacturer)	Portagen (Mead Johnson)	Pregestimil (Mead Johnson)	Pregestimil 24 (Mead Johnson)	Alimentum (Ross)	Nutramigen (Mead Johnson)
Calories/100 ml	67	67	81	67	67
Protein gm/100ml	2.3	1.8	2.2	1.8	1.8
Protein source	Sodium caseinate	Hydrolyzed casein w/added L-cystine, L-tyrosine & L-tryptophan	Hydrolyzed casein w/added L-cystine, L-tyrosine & L-tryptophan	Hydrolyzed casein w/added L-cystine, L-tyrosine & L-tryptophan	Hydrolyzed casein w/added L-cystine L-tryosine & L-tryptophan
CHO gm/100ml	7.6	6.8	8.0	6.8	7.3
CHO source	Corn syrup solids & sucrose	Corn syrup solids, dextrose, & modified corn starch	Corn syrup solids, dextrose, & modified corn starch	Sucrose & modified tapioca starch (70:30)	Corn syrup solids & modified corn starch
Fat gm/100ml	.2	3.7	4.4	3.6	3.3
Fat source	MCT & corn oils (86% MCT)	MCT, soy, corn, & high-oleic safflower oils (55:25:10:10)	MCT, soy, corn, & high-oleic safflower oils (55:25:10:10)	MCT, soy, & safflower oils (39:33:28)	Palm olein, soy, coconut, & high oleic sunflower oils (45:20:20:15)
Osmolality mOsm/kg	230	320	380	370	320
Sodium mEq (mg)/100ml	1.5 (36)	1.3 (31)	1.6 (37)	1.2 (29)	1.3 (31)
Potassium mEq (mg)/100ml	2.1 (83)	1.8 (73)	2.2 (87)	2.0 (78)	1.8 (73)
Calcium mEq (mg)/100ml	3.1 (62)	3.8 (76)	4.5 (91)	3.5 (70)	3.1 (62)
Phosphorus mEq(mg)/100ml	3.0 (46)	3.2 (50)	3.8 (59)	3.2 (50)	2.7 (42)
Iron mg/100ml	1.2	1.2	1.4	1.2	1.2
Notes:	For infants or children with impaired LCT fat digestion/ absorption	RTF hospital use only. Prepare from powder for home use.	For ↑ caloric demands and/or fluid restriction. RTF hospital use only. Prepare from powder for home use.		

TABLE 6 CONTINUED

Specialized Formulas for Infants

Elemental Formula: Crystalline Amino Acid Based

Product (Manufacturer)	Neocate (SHS)	Neocate 1+ (SHS)	Pediatric EO 28 (SHS)	EO28 EXTRA (SHS) unflavored	EleCare (Ross)	Vivonex Pediatric (Novartis)	Low Fat, High MCT Tolerex (Novartis)
Calories/100 ml	67	100	100	88.6	100	80	100
Protein gm/100ml	2.0	2.5	2.5	2.5	3.01	2.4	2.06
Protein source	L-amino acids	L-amino acids	L-amino acids	L- amino acids	L-amino acids	L-amino acids	L-amino acids
CHO gm/100ml	7.8	14.6	14.6	11.8	10.7	13.0	22.6
CHO source	Corn syrup solids	Corn syrup solids & sucrose	Maltodextrin & Sucrose	Dried glucose syrup*	Corn syrup solids	Maltodextrin & modified corn starch	Maltodextrin & modified corn starch
Fat gm/100ml	3.0	3.5	3.5	3.49	4.7	2.4	0.145
Fat source	Refined vegetable, hybrid safflower, coconut, & soy oils	Safflower, MCT, & canola oils	MCT, coconut, canola, & high-oleic safflower oils	Fractionated coconut, canola, & hybrid safflower oils (35:65)	High-oleic safflower, soy, & MCT oils (39:33:28)	MCT & soy oils	Safflower oil
Osmolality mOsm/kg	353	820 610*	820	636	596	360	550
Sodium mEq (mg)/100ml	1.0 (24)	.86 (20)	.9 (20)	2.6 (61)	2.0 (45)	1.7 (40)	2.0 (46.8)
Potassium mEq (mg)/100ml	2.6 (103)	2.3 (93)	3.3 (131)	2.3 (93.2)	3.8 (151)	3.1 (120)	3.0 (117)
Calcium mEq (mg)/100ml	4.1 (82)	3.1 (62)	3.1 (62)	37.5	5.4 (108)	4.8 (97)	55.6
Phosphorus mEq(mg)/100ml	4.0 (62)	4.0 (62)	4 (62)	40	5.2 (81)	5.1 (80)	55
Iron mg/100ml	1.2	.77	.8	.84	1.8	1.0	1.0
Notes:		*powder form	Formerly Neocate 1+ liquid	Powdered nutritionally complete elemental diet for adults with GI impairment and malabsorption			Only 1% total calories as linoleic that does not meet CON standards for infants.

TABLE 7

Pediatric Nutritionals

Product (Manufacturer)	Pediasure* (Ross)	Kindercal (Mead Johnson)	Pepdite One+ (SHS)	Resource Just for Kids (Novartis)	Peptamen Jr. (Ross)	Nutren Jr. (Nestle)
Calories/100 ml	100	106	100	100	100	100
Protein gm/100ml	3.0	3.4	3.1	3.0	3.0	3.0
Protein source	Sodium caseinate & whey protein concentrate	Sodium and calcium caseinate & milk protein concentrate (90:10)	L-amino acids & hydrolyzed protein (44:56)	Sodium and calcium caseinates & whey protein concentrate	Enzymatically hydrolyzed whey	Milk and whey protein
CHO gm/100ml	11	13.5	10.6	11.0	13.7	12.7
CHO source	Hydrolzed corn starch & sucrose (62:38)	Maltodextrin & sucrose (83:<17)	Corn syrup solids*	Hydrolyzed corn starch & sucrose*	Maltodextrin & corn starch*	Maltodextrin & sucrose
Fat gm/100ml	5.0	4.4	5.0	5.0	3.8	4.2
Fat source	High-oleic safflower, soy, & MCT oils (50:30:20)	Canola, high-oleic sunflower, corn, & MCT (50:15:15:20)	Fractionated coconut (MCT), canola, high-oleic safflower oils (35:65)	High-oleic sunflower, soy & MCT oils	MCT, soy, canola, & soy lecithin oils MCT:LCT 60:40	Soybean, MCT, canola & soy lecithin
Osmolality mOsm/kg	335 *345 w/fiber	310	430	390 (440*)	260-360	25:75
Sodium mEq (mg)/100ml	1.65 (38)	1.6 (37)	1.78 (41)	2.6 (59)	2.0 (46)	350
Potassium mEq (mg)/100ml	3.3 (131)	3.3 (131)	3.4 (136)	2.9 (114)	3.3 (132)	2.0 (46)
Calcium mEq (mg)/100ml	4.8 (97)	4.2 (85)	5.6 (113)	5.7 (114)	5.0 (100)	3.3 (132)
Phosphorus mEq(mg)/100ml	5.3 (80)	5.4 (85)	6.0 (94)	5.1 (80)	5.3 (80)	5.0 (100)
Iron mg/100ml	1.39	1.0	1.4	1.4	1.4	5.1 (80)
Notes:	*w/fiber= .5g/100ml		Flavored product contains surcrose	French Vanilla flavor *chocolate	*flavored oral products contain sucrose	1.4

TABLE 8

Adult Nutritionals

Product (Manufacturer)	Peptamen with FOS/ Inulin* (Nestle)	Peptamen 1.5 (Nestle)	Peptamen VHP (Nestle)	Nutren 1.5 (Nestle)	Nutren 2.0 (Nestle)	Boost (Mead Johnson)Vanilla Flavor	Nepro (Ross) Vanilla	Vital HN (Ross)	EO28 EXTRA (SHS) unflavored
Calories/100 ml	100	150	100	150	200	101	200	100	88.6
Protein gm/100ml	4.0	6.7	6.2	6.0	8.0	15.8	7.0	4.1	2.5
Protein source	Enzymatically hydrolyzed whey	Enzymatically hydrolyzed whey	Enzymatically hydrolyzed whey	Calcium-Potassium caseinate	Calcium-Potassium caseinate	Milk protein concentrate	Calcium, magnesium, & Sodium caseinates	Whey, meat and soy protein, & free amino acids	L- amino acids
CHO gm/100ml	12.4	18.7	10.4	16.9	19.6	17.3	22.2	18.5	11.8
CHO source	Maltodextrin & corn starch	Maltodextrin & corn starch*	Maltodextrin & corn starch*	Maltodextrin*	Corn syrup solids, maltodextrin, & sucrose	Corn syrup solids & sugar	Corn syrup & sucrose	Maltodextrin & sucrose	Dried glucose syrup*
Fat gm/100ml	3.9	5.5	3.9	6.7	10.6	1.76	9.5	1.0	3.49
Fat source	MCT, soy, & soy lecithin oils MCT: LCT 70:30	MCT, soy, & soy lecithin oils MCT: LCT 70:30	MCT, soy, & soy lecithin oils MCT: LCT 70:30	MCT, canola, corn, & soy lecithin oils MCT: LCT 50:50	MCT, canola, soy lecithin, & corn oils, MCT:LCT 75:25	Canola, high-oleic sunflower & corn oil	High-oleic safflower, canola, & soy lecithin oils	Safflower & MCT oils	Fractionated coconut, canola &hybrid safflower oils (35:65)
Osmolality mOsm/kg	290	550	300 to 430**	510	745	610 to 670	665	500	636
Sodium mEq (mg)/100ml	2.4 (56)	4.3 (102)	2.4 (560)	5.0 (116)	5.6 (130)	2.4 (55)	3.6 (84.5)	2.4 (56.6)	2.6 (61)
Potassium mEq (mg)/100ml	3.8 (150)	4.8 (186)	3.8 (150)	4.8 (187)	4.9 (192)	4.3 (169)	2.7 (106)	3.5 (140)	2.3 (93.2)
Calcium mEq (mg)/100ml	4.0 (80)	5.0 (100)	4.0 (80)	5.0 (100)	6.7 (134)	137	137	66.7	37.5
Phosphorus mEq(mg)/100ml	4.5 (70)	6.4 (100)	4.5 (70)	6.4 (100)	8.6 (134)	132	68.5	66.7	40
Iron mg/100ml	1.8	2.7	1.8	1.8	2.4	1.9	1.9	1.2	.84
Notes:	*fiber source FOS Inulin 4gm/1000ml	*Flavored product contains sucrose	*flavored product contains sucrose **range for flavors	*Flavored product contains sucrose		Complete oral supplement	Complete, balanced protein for people on dialysis	Nutritionally complete, partially hydrolyzed diet for patients with gastrointestinal function (maldigestion, malabsorption)	Powdered nutritionally complete elemental diet for adults with malabsorption and impairment of the GI tract.

TABLE 9

Modulars

Product (Manufacturer)	Protein-Free: Product 80056 (Mead Johnson) per 100 gm	Pro-Phree (Ross) per 100 gm	Super Soluble Duocal (SHS) per 100 gm	Carbohydrate-Free: Product 3232 (Mead Johnson) per 100gm	ARCF (Ross) 100 ml
Calories/100 ml	495	510	490	517	81
Protein gm/100ml	0	0	0	22	4.0
Protein source	--	--	--	Casein hydrolysates and free amino acids	Soy protein isolate
CHO gm/100ml	72	65	73	33	0
CHO source	Corn syrup solids & modified tapioca starch	Corn syrup solids	Hydrolyzed corn starch	Modified tapioca starch	--
Fat gm/100ml	23	28	22	33	4.0
Fat source	Corn oil	High-oleic safflower, coconut & soy oils	Blend of refined vegetable (corn, coconut) & MCT oils	MCT, corn & soy lecithin oils	High-oleic safflower, coconut & soy oils (40:30:30)
Sodium mEq (mg)/100ml	3.1 (72)	11 (250)	.9 (<20)	14.7 (340)	2.6 (59)
Potassium mEq (mg)/100ml	8.7 (340)	22 (875)	.1 (<5)	22 (860)	3.7 (146)
Calcium mEq (mg)/100ml	540	750	<5	740	140
Phosphorus mEq(mg)/100ml	300	525	<5	490	100
Iron mg/100ml	10.8	11.9	--	14.8	2.4
Notes:	Protein-free formula base for use with added protein, sodium, potassium and chloride. Indicated for individuals requiring specific mixtures of amino acids.	Protein-free energy module. Nutrition support of infants and toddlers requiring reduced protein intake, specific mixture of l-amino acids or increased energy, minerals and vitamins.	High-calorie, protein-free, lactose-free and gluten-free. 1 Tbsp. =8.5gm Duocal = 42 cal.	Mono- & disaccharide-free powder. Used in the identification and dietary management of disaccharide deficiencies or impaired glucose transport, & intractable diarrhea.	Indicated for those unable to tolerate type or amount of CHO in standard formulas.

TABLE 10

Nutritional Modulars and Additives

Product (Manufacturer)	Polycose Liquid 100 ml (Ross)	Polycose Powder 100gm (Ross)	Promod Powder one 6.6gm scoop (Ross)	Corn oil	Microlipid analysis per 89ml bottle (Mead Johnson)	MCT oil (Mead Johnson)	Casec Powder per Tbsp. = 4.4gm (Mead Johnson)	Instant Nonfat Dry Milk Powder	Carnation Instant Breakfast Mix vanilla crème (Nestle) 1.26 oz pkg/36gm	Cow and Goat Milk: Nonfat Milk	2% Lowfat Milk	Whole Milk	Goat Milk
Calories/100 ml	200 (1ml=2cal)	380 (3.8/gm*)	28 (4.2/gm*)	8.4/ml	400 (4.5/ml)	8.3/gm or 7.7/ml	17	3.5/gm	130	35.8	51.5	67	68.8
Protein gm/100ml	--	--	5.5	--	--	--	4 (.9/gm)	.35	5.0	3.5	3.4	3.5	3.5
Protein source	--	--	Whey protein concentrate	--	--	--	Calcium caseinate	Cow's milk	Nonfat dry milk	Cow's milk	Cow's milk	Cow's milk	Goat's milk
CHO gm/100ml	50	94	0.67	--	--	--	--	.52	28	4.9	4.9	4.9	4.4
CHO source	Glucose polymers	Glucose polymers	--	--	--	--	--	Lactose	Maltodextrin, sugar, & lactose	Lactose	Lactose	lactose	Lactose
Fat gm/100ml	--	--	0.60	15g/Tbsp.	45	8.3	.09	--	--	.01	1.9	3.5	4.1
Fat source	--	--	Soy lecithin	Corn	Safflower oil	MCT	Soy lecithin	--	--	Butterfat	Butterfat	Butterfat	Butterfat
Osmolality mOsm/kg	900	900 in solution	30/scoop	-	-	-	-	-	-	-	-	-	-
Sodium mEq (mg)/100ml	3.0 (70)	4.8 (110)	1.09 (25)	--	--	--	.19 (4.4)	.23 (5.3)	4.5 (105)	2.2 (52.5)	2.2 (51.5)	2.2 (51)	2.1 (51)
Potassium mEq (mg)/100ml	.15 (6)	.3 (10)	1.15 (45)	--	--	--	.01 (.44)	.45 (17.9)	6.1 (240)	4.3 (169)	4.0 (158)	3.9 (154)	5.2 (204)
Calcium mEq (mg)/100ml	1.0 (20)	1.5 (30)	3.24 (65)	--	--	--	3.1 (62)	12.5	--	125	125	123	133
Phosphorus mEq(mg)/100ml	.19 (3)	.77 (12)	2.1 (33)	--	--	--	2.2 (35)	9.6	--	103	97.9	96	110
Iron mg/100ml	--	--	--	--	--	--	--	--	--	.04	.05	trace	.05
Notes:		*1 tsp.= 2g=8 cals 1 tbsp.= =23 cals ¼ C.=25g =95cals	*1scoop= 6.6g 6g=1.3g 1tbsp=4g	%linoleic from fat: 58%	1tbsp =5.9g Linoleic acid	f.a.% <C8 <6 C8 67 C10 27 >C10 <4							

TABLE 11

Pediatric Metabolic Formulas: PKU

Product (Manufacturer)	Lofenalac (Mead Johnsom) per 100 gm	Phenyl-Free 1 (Mead Johnson) per 100 gm	Phenyl-Free 2 (Mead Johnson) per 100 gm	Phenyl-Free 2HP (Mead Johnson) per 100 gm	Phenex-1 (Ross) per 100 gm	Xphe Analog (SHS) per 100gm	XP Maxamaid (SHS) per 100 gm
Calories/100 ml	462	500	410	390	480	475	350
Protein gm/100ml	15	16.2	22	40	15	13	25
Protein source	Specially treated hydrolysates & L-amino acids	L-amino acids	L-amino acids	L-amino acids	L-amino acids	L-amino acids	L-amino acids
CHO gm/100ml	60	51	60	44	53	59	62
CHO source	Corn syrup solids & modified tapioca starch	Corn syrup solids, modified corn starch, & sucrose	Sucrose, corn syrup solids, & modified corn starch	Sucrose, corn syrup solids, & modified corn starch	Corn syrup solids	Corn syrup solids	Corn syrup solids
Fat gm/100ml	18	26	8.6	6.3	21.7	20.9	--
Fat source	Corn oil	Palm-olein, soy, coconut, & high-oleic sunflower oils	Soy oil	Soy oil	High-oleic safflower, coconut, & soy oils	Refined animal fat, peanut, & coconut oil	--
Sodium mEq (mg)/100ml	9.5 (220)	10.4 (240)	27 (610)	18 (410)	8 (190)	5.2 (120)	25 (580)
Potassium mEq (mg)/100ml	12 (470)	14.3 (560)	28 (1100)	30 (1180)	17 (675)	10.8 (420)	22 (840)
Calcium mEq (mg)/100ml	430	660	980	730	575	600	810
Phosphorus mEq(mg)/100ml	320	440	980	730	400	500	810
Iron mg/100ml	8.7	9.6	12.2	15.7	9	10	12
Notes:	Low phenylalanine diet powder for infants and children w/hyper-phenylalaninemia including PKU Phe = 75 gm per 100 gm powder	Phenylalanine-free diet powder for mgt of infants and toddlers with PKU. Important to provide enough Phe using other foods to support growth.	Phenylalanine-free powder for children and adults with PKU.	Phenylalanine-free powder for children and adults with PKU. High protein levels for maternal PKU or individuals with calorie and volume restriction.	Phenylalanine-free powder for infants and toddlers with PKU. Must be supplemented with intact protein to meet Phe requirements and support growth.	Unflavored, phenylalanine-free powdered infant formula Must be consumed in conjunction w/whole protein source (breast milk or infant formula) to meet phenylalanine requirements and ensure normal growth	Phenylalanine-free powdered formula used in mgt of PKU in children 1-8 yrs. Available in orange and unflavored. Fat, CHO, and low protein sources may be used to supply the remainder of calories and to fulfill the EFA

TABLE 12

Pediatric Metabolic Formulas: Maple Syrup Urine Disease (MSUD) & Urea Cycle Disorders

Product (Manufacturer)	BCAD 2 (Mead Johnson) per 100 gm	Cyclinex-1 (Ross) per 100 gm	Cyclinex-2 (Ross) per 100 gm	Ketonex 1 (Ross) per 100 gm	Ketonex 2 (Ross) per 100 gm	MSUD Analog (SHS) per 100 gm	MSUD Maxamaid (SHS) per 100 gm	MSUD Diet Powder (Mead Johnson) per 100 gm
Calories/100 ml	410	510	440	480	410	475	350	464
Protein gm/100ml	24	7.5	15	15	30	13	25	8.1
Protein source	L-amino acids	L-amino acids	L-amino acids	L-amino acids	L-amino acids	L-amino acids	L-amino acids	L amino acids
CHO gm/100ml	57	57	45	53	35	59	62	63
CHO source	Corn syrup solids, sugar, & modified corn starch	Corn syrup solids	Corn syrup solids	Corn syrup solids	Corn syrup solids	Corn syrup solids	Sucrose & corn syrup solids	Corn syrup solids & modified tapioca starch
Fat gm/100ml	8.5	24.6	17	21.7	14	20.9	<0.5	20
Fat source	Soy oil	High-oleic safflower, coconut, & soy oils	High-oleic safflower, coconut, & soy oils	High-oleic safflower, coconut, & soy oils	High-oleic safflower, coconut, & soy oils	Peanut, coconut, & refined animal fat (pork)	--	Corn oil
Sodium mEq (mg)/100ml	26.5 (610)	9 (215)	51 (1175)	8 (190)	38 (880)	5.2 (120)	25 (580)	8 (184)
Potassium mEq (mg)/100ml	31.2 (1220)	20 (760)	46 (1800)	17 (675)	35 (1370)	10.8 (420)	22 (840)	12.5 (490)
Calcium mEq (mg)/100ml	730	650	1150	575	880	600	810	490
Phosphorus mEq(mg)/100ml	730	455	1020	400	760	500	810	260
Iron mg/100ml	12.2	17	17	9	13	10	12	8.9
Notes:	Diet powder used for the dietary mgt of children and adults with MSUD or other inborn errors of branched chain amino acid metabolism of BCAD stands for branched chain amino acid disorder	Amino acid modified medical food. Nutrition support of infants and toddlers with a urea cycle disorder, gyrate atrophy the choroids and retina, or HHH syndrome.	Amino acid modified medical food. Nutrition support of children and adults with a urea cycle disorder, gyrate atrophy of the choroids and retina, or HHH syndrome.	Amino acid modified medical food for infants and toddlers with MSUD & B ketothiolase deficiency	Amino acid modified medical food For children and adults with MSUD or beta-ketothiolase deficiency.	Unflavored, iso-leucine-, leucine- & valine-free. Must be used with a whole protein source (breast milk or infant formula) in quantities to meet isoleucine, leucine & valine requirements and ensure normal growth.	Orange flavored, valine-, leucine-, & isoleucine-free powdered food used in the mgt of MSUD in children aged 1 to 8 years	Diet powder with no leucine, isoleucine, or valine. For the mgt. Of infants and children with disorders of branched chain amino acid metabolism including MSUD

TABLE 13

Pediatric Metabolic Formulas: Organic Acidemia

Product (Manufacturer)	OS 1 (Mead Johnson) per 100 gm	OS 2 (Mead Johnson) per 100 gm	Propimex-1 (Ross) per 100 gm	Propimex-2 (Ross) per 100 gm	Xphe, Xtyr Anaog (SHS) per 100 gm	Xphe Tyr Maxamaid (SHS) per 100 gm	Tyrosinemia Type 1 XPTM Analog (SHS) per 100 gm	Tyros 2 (Mead Johnson) per 100 gm
Calories/100 ml	280	300	480	410	475	350	475	410
Protein gm/100ml	42	56	15	30	13	25	13	22
Protein source	L-amino acids	L-amino acids	L-amino acids	L-amino acids	L-amino acids	L-amino acids	l-amino acids	Amino acids
CHO gm/100ml	27	19	53	35	59	62	59	60
CHO source	Sucrose	Sucrose	Corn syrup solids	Corn syrup solids	Corn syrup solids	Corn syrup solids & sucrose	Corn syrup solids	Corn syrup solids, sugar, & modified corn starch
Fat gm/100ml	0	0	21.7	13	20.9	<0.5	20.9	8.5
Fat source	--	--	High-oleic safflower, coconut, & soy oils	High-oleic safflower, coconut, & soy oils	Safflower, coconut, & soy oils	--	Safflower, coconut, & soy oils	Soy oil
Sodium mEq (mg)/100ml	47 (1070)	28 (640)	8 (190)	38 (880)	5.2 (120)	25 (580)	5.2 (120)	27 (610)
Potassium mEq (mg)/100ml	59 (2300)	34 (1330)	17 (675)	35 (1370)	10.8 (420)	22 (840)	10.8 (420)	28 (1100)
Calcium mEq (mg)/100ml	2400	1310	575	880	600	810	600	730
Phosphorus mEq(mg)/100ml	1860	1010	400	760	500	810	500	730
Iron mg/100ml	34	15	9	13	10	12	8	12.2
Notes:	Amino acid modified powder. Used for infants with propionic or methylmalonic academia. Isoleucine-, methionine-, threonine- and valine-free. May contain 100mg ILE/ 100gm.	Amino acid modified powder. Used for children with propionic or methylmalonic academia. Isoleucine, methionine- threonine- and valine-free.	Amino acid modified medical food. Nutrition support of infants and toddlers with propionic or methylmalonic academia. Methionine- and valine-free and low in isoleucine, threonine and tryptophan.	Amino acid modified medical food. Nutrition support of children and adults with propionic or methyl malonic academia. Methionine- and valine-free. Low in isoleuc ine, threonine and tryptophan.	Unflavored phenylalanine- & tyrosine-free powdered infant formula for mgt of tyrosinemia when plasma methionine levels are normal.	Orange flavored phenylalanine & tyrosine free powdered medical food. with tyrosinemia aged 1 to 8 years.	Unflavored, phenylalanine-tyrosine- & methionine-free powdered infant formula. For infants with tyrosinemia type 1.	Used for dietary management of children and adults with tyrosinemia type II or other inborn errors of tyrosine metabolism. Phenylalanine- & Tyrosine-free.

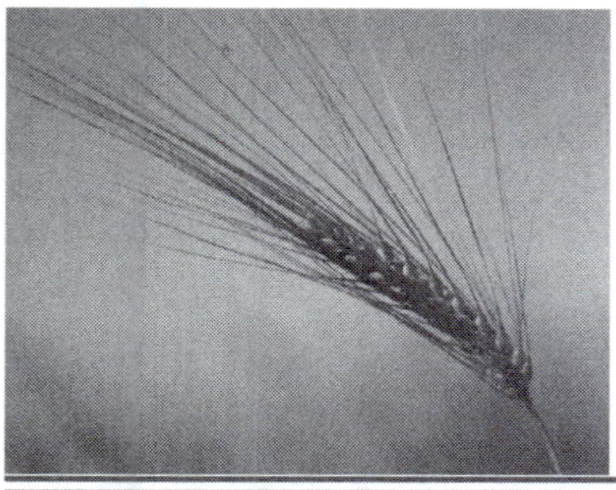

Index

Build Your Library

Along with this title, we publish numerous products on a variety of topics. We are sure that you will find the below titles to be an essential addition to your library. Order your copies today or contact us for a copy of our latest catalog for additional product information.

Practical Nutritional Support Techniques, Second Edition

Alan L. Buchman, MD, MSPH

224 pp., Soft Cover, 2003, ISBN 1-55642-628-3, Order #76283, **$37.95**

The perfect reference for the management of patients that require nutritional support. Organized in a "how-to" approach, everyone connected with the field of GI will appreciate the ease and applicability it will bring to their professions. Inside these easy-to-read chapters you will find how to determine "why, how much, what type, and how to monitor" these therapies. Also inside you will find practical tables, figures, algorithms, and bibliographies.

The Clinician's Guide to Inflammatory Bowel Disease

Gary R. Lichtenstein, MD

336 pp., Soft Cover, 2003, ISBN 1-55642-554-6, Order #75546, **$44.95**

This valuable resource is a user-friendly, quick reference manual on inflammatory bowel disease. Inside this state-of-the-art guide, you will find line drawings and photos, tables, algorithms, and bulleted text with key facts. An essential resource for gastroenterologists, medical students, fellows, internists, and family practitioners.

Office Gastroenterology: Life Made Simple

Isaac Raijman, MD

250 pp., Soft Cover, 2004, ISBN 1-55642-610-0, Order #76100, **$99.95**

In a language that is user friendly and easy to understand, today's common gastroenterology problems are explained in a variety of ways, such as how often they occur, the symptoms they produce, the significance of the disease, and how to diagnose them. A perfect resource for office personnel, general practitioners, students, and patients who want to better understand health problems.

Contact Us

SLACK Incorporated, Professional Book Division
6900 Grove Road, Thorofare, NJ 08086
1-800-257-8290/1-856-848-1000, Fax: 1-856-853-5991
orders@slackinc.com or www.slackbooks.com

Order Form

Quantity	Title	Order #	Price
	Practical Nutritional Support Techniques	76283	**$37.95**
	The Clinician's Guide to Inflammatory Bowel Disease	75546	**$44.95**
	Office Gastroenterology: Life Made Simple	76100	**$99.95**

Subtotal	$
Applicable state and local tax will be added to your purchase	$
Handling	**$4.50**
Total	$

Name: ____________________
Address: ____________________
City: __________ State: ______ Zip: ______
Phone: __________ Fax: __________
Email: ____________________

- Check enclosed (Payable to SLACK Incorporated)______
- Charge my: ___ MasterCard ___ VISA ___

Account #: ____________________
Exp. date: ________ Signature: ____________________

***NOTE:** Prices are subject to change without notice. Shipping charges will apply. Shipping and handling charges are non-refundable.*

CODE: 328